CAREGIVER'S COMPASS

MASTERING THE ART OF COMPASSIONATE DEMENTIA CAREGIVING

ALEX J BUISON

Author: ALEX J BUISON

Title: CAREGIVER'S COMPASS

ISBN: 978-1-965615-81-2

Category: SELF-HELP/Personal Growth/Caregiving/Health/Success

Publisher: Caregivers Today, LLC

Address: 9107 Mount Wilson Street, Las Vegas, Nevada, USA 89113 Website: www.caregiverstoday.org

....

DEDICATION

To my beloved parents, Edgardo and Gloria Buison, Every step I've taken toward my dreams has been possible because of your love, patience, and strength.

This book is a small offering for the endless gifts you've given me.

With deepest love and gratitude,

Your son, Alex J Buison

ACKNOWLEDGMENTS

First of all, I would like to thank you all for taking the time to focus on being the best caregiver you could possibly become by taking the time to find helpful resources that are available to you on your personal caregiving journey. To my wife, Lyn—my soulmate and constant anchor. Your love and unwavering support make everything possible. To my grandparents, whose compassion and wisdom inspired my journey—you gave me purpose and a heart for caregiving. To my sister, Maria, and my brother, Eric—your encouragement and faith in me have been my greatest blessings. This book exists because of your love and belief in me. Thank you from the bottom of my heart!

I would like to give a special salute to all the nurses in the world and to all that I have been associated with in my journey working in the healthcare field. These people are the true heroes with the hearts of angels when it comes to providing the best care for everyone and providing assistance to those who may be ill and the elderly, who deserve the proper care in their time of need.

Of course, I need to mention all my family and friends who have been there for me and supported me through all of my life experiences, whether they were happy or sad. A special thanks to everyone, and may God bless all of you.

Finally, to my dear friend and mentor Gerry Robert and his awesome team, who have helped me with publishing and making this book a reality. I hope this will be the start of my support for all caregivers in the world.

Table of Contents

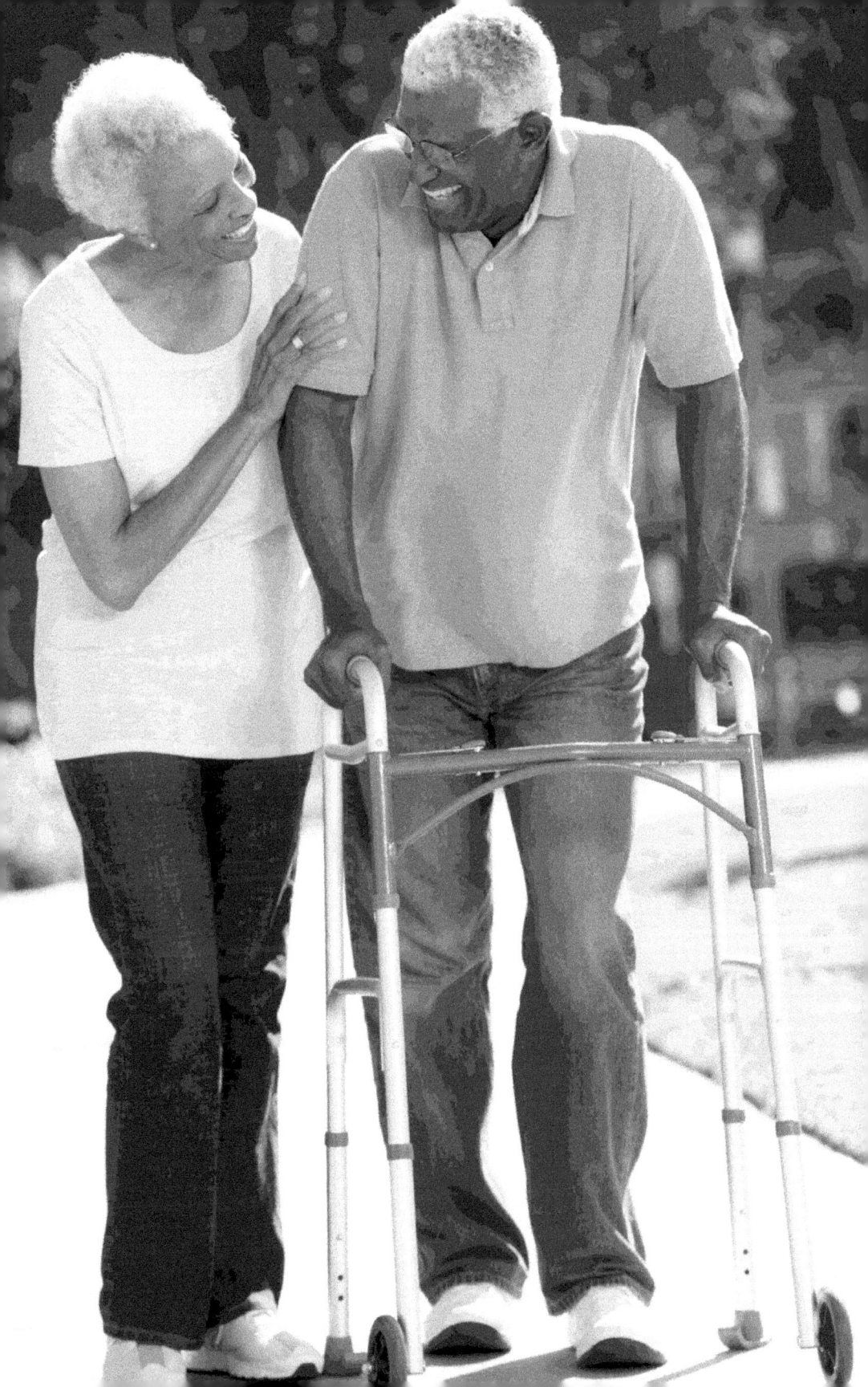

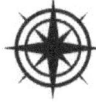

Chapter One.
Embracing the Journey of Caregiving

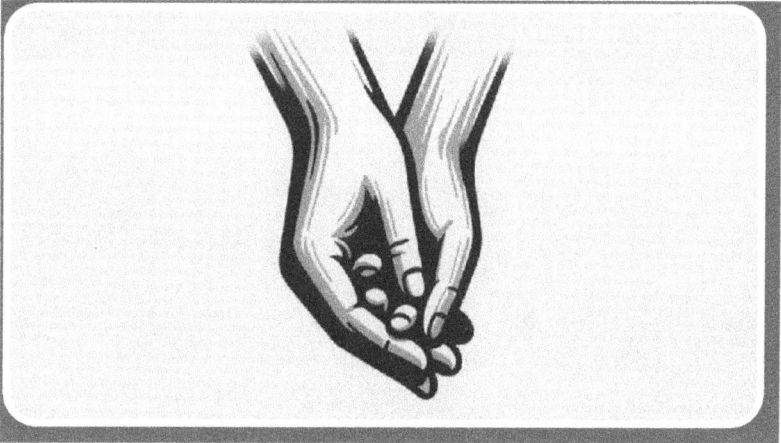

"One person caring about another represents life's Greatest Value."

– Jim Rohn

Caregiving for someone with dementia is like stepping onto a path that twists and turns in unexpected ways. It's a role that asks much of you, often changing from moment to moment.

One minute you're a helper, and the next one you're a guide. You're the keeper of stories, the protector of dignity, and sometimes you're the closest thing to a memory that person can reach. This role is complex. It's not just a list of tasks but a weave of emotional, physical, and sometimes spiritual support. Why is it complex? Because people are complex. Dementia patients experience the world differently, with their memories fading and their sense of reality shifting. As their caregiver, you must adapt, learn, and grow to meet their ever-changing needs. You become a student of patience, a master of creativity, and a warrior of compassion.

And why does it matter so much that you do this well? Because proper care can make all the difference. Not just for the person with dementia, but for you as well. Good caregiving can bring comfort and joy to days that might otherwise be filled with confusion and sadness. It can create moments of connection that remind the person they are loved and not alone in their journey.

When you care for someone with dementia, you're doing more than just helping them get through the day. You're supporting their mind, their heart, and their spirit. This is why effective caregiving matters so much. It's about ensuring safety, yes, but it's also about nurturing the person's sense of self. It's about creating a space where they can feel understood and respected, despite the challenges dementia brings.

But let's not forget about you, the caregiver. Your well-being is just as important. When you learn to provide care effectively, you also learn to take care of yourself. You find balance. You discover ways to recharge, to find joy in your own life, and to build resilience.

Why? Because you cannot pour from an empty cup. Taking care of yourself allows you to give the best care to others. Taking this step—the step you're taking right now—is something to celebrate. It shows courage. It shows love. And it shows a commitment to making life better, both for the person with dementia you're caring for and for yourself.

You've decided to seek knowledge, to learn, and to grow. By doing this, you're preparing to face the challenges of dementia care with new tools, a new understanding, and a renewed heart. You're not just reading words on a page. You're joining a community of caregivers who share your journey, who understand your struggles, and who are cheering you on.

This book is your guide. It's filled with the information you need to improve your skills and approach caregiving with confidence and compassion. And as you turn each page, remember that you're taking a step toward a better, more fulfilling experience for both you and the person you care for. You're about to embark on a profound exploration into the world of caregiving for dementia patients. This journey is a transformative one, with challenges and triumphs alike. It's a path that will teach you about the depths of human connection, the strength of your spirit, and the incredible impact of caring for another. Welcome to the journey. Welcome to a new chapter in your life as a caregiver.

My Story: Alex J Buison's Path to Compassionate Care

Hello. My name is Alex J Buison. I want to share with you a journey—a deeply personal story that, in many ways, may resonate with your own experiences as a caregiver. My story is not just about the path I've taken in my career but about how life's challenges have shaped me into the caregiver I am today.

Picture a young boy arriving in the United States at the tender age of eight. This boy, born in the Philippines, landed in Michigan with a mix of hope and uncertainty in his heart. That boy was me. I remember the cold winters, so different from the tropical warmth of my birth country. I remember feeling both lost and found in this new world. But what stood out the most was a deep sense of care from the people around me—something that would define my life's calling.

A tragedy struck early in my life when my mother passed away. I was only ten years old. Her absence left a gaping hole in my heart, one that could only be filled with the love and care of my grandparents. They became my guardians, my mentors, and my pillars of strength. My father, industrious and caring, worked tirelessly to provide for us. But it was in the warmth of my grandparents' care that I discovered my true purpose: to serve, nurture, and care for those in the twilight of their lives.

My academic path started with a fascination for the human body. I pursued a degree in biochemistry at the University of Michigan-Dearborn, which further fueled my curiosity. Yet, amidst the molecules and reactions, I found that my heart yearned for a more direct way to impact lives. This led me to Wayne State University, where I earned a Bachelor of Nursing. Here, I learned not just the science of medicine but also the art of healing through compassion and empathy.

Over the past 25 years, I've dedicated my life to nursing. I've traversed the country as a cardiac unit travel nurse, absorbing diverse cultures and medical practices.

But it was in the field of Hospice and Gerontology Care where I found my true calling. It is here, in the quiet rooms and the gentle goodbyes, that I learned the most valuable lessons about life and care.

Caregiving, I've learned, is not just about medical expertise. It's about a connection, a shared moment of understanding, a gentle touch, and a listening ear. My Filipino-American heritage plays a vital role in my approach to care. We Filipinos value family, respect for elders, and a strong sense of community. These values are deeply ingrained in me and guide my hands and heart as I provide care.

But the journey has not been without challenges. Caregiver stress and burnout are very real and can take a heavy toll. I've seen it in my colleagues and felt it within myself. It pushed me to search for resilience strategies, not just for my own benefit but to share with fellow caregivers. It's not just about enduring; it's about thriving in the role we've embraced.

Self-care is paramount. The act of caring for others must not overshadow the care we owe ourselves. This understanding led me to focus on training other caregivers. Providing them with the tools to be compassionate and empathetic is as important as any medical procedure. It is my mission to help caregivers navigate the complex emotional landscape of our work, preventing burnout and promoting a culture of resilient caregiving.

In the coming months, I'm excited to launch a new beginning. I'll be starting locally in Las Vegas, Nevada, focusing on giving the best care and support to caregivers. The goal is to scale this nationwide and, eventually, worldwide. It's about creating a community, a network of caregivers who can support and uplift each other. My work is more than a job; it's a commitment to honor the legacy of those who cared for me. It's about passing the torch, spreading knowledge, and empowering every caregiver to provide the best possible care.

This is my story, my path to compassionate care. And this story is just the beginning. What follows in this book is an exploration of the skills and techniques that have not only helped me but countless others in the caregiving field. We will dive deep into practical, actionable advice that goes beyond the pages, influencing your daily life and the lives you touch. Together, we will embark on this transformative journey.

As we move forward, remember that you are not alone. We are part of a grand community, a family of caregivers united by our dedication and love for those we serve. I invite you to join me, to learn from my experiences, and to build upon them. Together, we will redefine what it means to care and in doing so, find a deeper understanding of our purpose and joy in our service.

Welcome to our community, and let's begin this journey of compassionate caregiving together.

The Caregiver's Transformation

Caregiving is a path walked with love, patience, and an open heart. You are here because you care. You're here because you want to make a difference in the life of someone with dementia. Your choice to step into the role of a caregiver is brave and kind. And I want to tell you, that your journey is valued. This book is a friend on your journey; it is here to guide you with skills and techniques you can use every day. It's full of ideas that will help you and the person you care for. I have taken care to make sure these pages speak to you, to make sure they are clear and full of advice you can put to work right away.

What will you learn? You will learn how to understand what a person with dementia might feel and need. Every chapter will give you new tools. These tools will help you create a calm and loving space for the person you care for. You will find ways to talk and listen that bring you closer. You will learn how to handle hard moments with kindness and how to take care of yourself too. This book is different. It is just for you, the caregiver of someone with dementia. It knows the hard work you do. It shows the love you give. And it is here to help you give care that makes life better for you and the person you are helping. When you use what you learn, you will see change. The person you care for will feel safer and happier. And you? You will find strength and peace in your caregiving. Your days might become lighter. Your heart might feel more joy. As you turn each page, you will see that you are not alone. There are many caregivers like you. And together, with this book in hand, you can bring more love and care to those who need it the most. Join me on this path. Let's walk it together. Let's learn and grow. Let's make each day a little brighter for you and for those you care for. This is your caregiver's transformation.

Navigating the Chapters

You've opened a door to a world that's both challenging and rewarding. The world of caregiving for those with dementia is one that requires patience, love, and a deep sense of understanding. This book is your map of that world.

Now, let me guide you through each chapter of this book. Picture it as a journey we're about to embark on together. A journey where each step, each chapter, brings us closer to the heart of compassionate caregiving. Let's step forward. Each chapter in this book has been crafted to build upon the last. Like the base of a mountain, we begin with a strong foundation. The chapters progress, each one a stepping stone, leading to the peak of caregiving mastery. You're not just flipping through pages; you're climbing towards a summit of knowledge and understanding.

At the heart of this book is the EMPATHIZE framework. This framework is like a compass, guiding you on your journey. It aligns perfectly with my 9-Step

Calm Caregiving Course. Each letter in EMPATHIZE stands for one of the vital traits or skills you'll develop as a caregiver and has a chapter dedicated to it. We'll explore this framework in more detail as we move through the book, but know that it's there to keep you on track and to ensure that no step is taken in vain.

Encounter with Dementia: Chapter 2

Mindfulness in Caregiving: Chapter 3

Patience with Progress: Chapter 4

Adaptability in Caregiving: Chapter 5

Tenderness in Dementia Care: Chapter 6

Holistic Care Strategies: Chapter 7

Inspiration for Caregivers: Chapter 8

Zeal for Caregiving: Chapter 9

Empowerment Through Knowledge: Chapter 10

Our first chapter is about embracing caregiving. Here, we lay the groundwork for the path ahead. Understanding the role of a caregiver is crucial. It's the soil from which all the care you give will grow. We'll talk about why this role is so complex and why your job is so vital, not just for the ones you care for but for you as well.

Following that, you'll walk with me through my journey. Stories have a way of carrying lessons deep into our hearts. My story is no different. It's a tale of loss, of finding a calling in eldercare and hospice nursing, and of how my Filipino-American heritage shaped my approach to care. It's a personal narrative, sure, but within it are universal truths that can help fortify you on your caregiving journey.

Then, we'll delve into the transformation that caregiving can bring about. You're not just changing the lives of those you care for; you're evolving too. This book will show you skills and techniques that can reshape the way you approach caregiving. And, most importantly, how these changes can improve your quality of life as well as that of the person you're caring for.

The chapters that follow are each dedicated to a specific aspect of the EMPATHIZE framework. From establishing meaningful connections to handling difficult emotions — both yours and your loved one's. We'll cover practical strategies for managing the day-to-day challenges of dementia caregiving. Each strategy is a tool for your toolkit, something you can use right away to make a real difference.

As you move through these chapters, you'll find that they're more than just informational. They're a call to action. They're your opportunity to engage with the material, to take what you learn and apply it directly to your caregiving situation. Every piece of advice is actionable and meant to be put into practice.

Moreover, this book is not just a solitary journey. It's a community. By reading it, you're joining a group of people all dedicated to the art of caregiving. And, as you learn and grow, you'll find that the book is just the beginning. Our online resources, courses, and counseling services are there to support you further. We encourage you to join our community, subscribe to our newsletter, and follow the learning resources we provide. They're all designed to give you continued guidance and support.

By the time you reach the final chapter, you have read more than just a book. You have undergone a transformation. You'll see things differently, approach situations uniquely, and have a toolkit filled with effective strategies. The transformation is not just in the knowledge you gain but in the actions you take and the changes you make.

So, take your time with each chapter. Read slowly, reflect, and engage with the exercises. Use the resources we offer to deepen your understanding. Remember, this isn't just about reading; it's about changing lives — yours and those of the people you care for. Welcome to the journey of a lifetime. Let's begin.

Chapter Two.
Encounter with Dementia

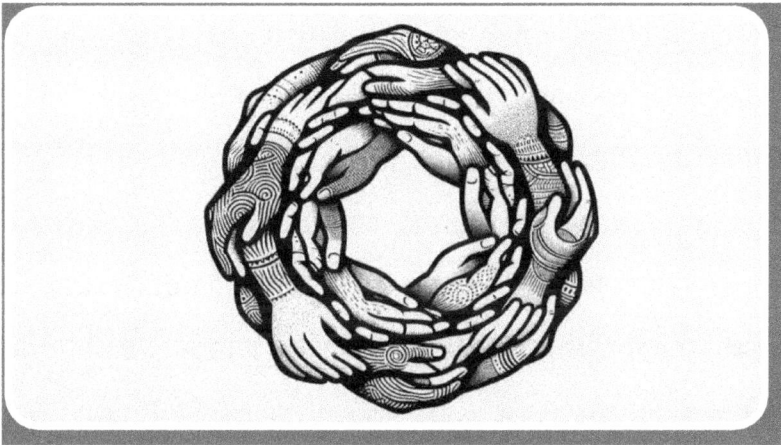

"Those with dementia may have a brain that works much differently than ours, but if we link our hands together we can overcome anything."

– Teepa Snow

Understanding Dementia and Setting Expectations

Dementia is a word that we hear a lot, but what does it mean? Let's talk about it. Dementia is not just one thing. It is a group of symptoms that affect a person's memory, their ability to do things, and how they understand the world around them. It's like when a person starts forgetting the names of their friends or how to go home from the store. This can be hard, not just for the person with dementia but for their family and friends too.

When someone finds out that a family member has dementia, it can be a shock. You might not know what to do or how to feel. That's normal. It's a big change. But there are things you can do to make it better, both for you and for the person with dementia.

The first step is to set expectations. This means understanding that dementia will change things. The person with dementia will change. They might forget more or get confused more easily. They might not seem like the same person sometimes. It's hard, but knowing this can help you get ready for what's coming. You can learn how to help them and how to take care of yourself too.

Now, let's take a little time to talk about why setting expectations is so important. When we expect something, we can plan for it. If you know it might rain, you should bring an umbrella, right? It's the same with dementia care. If you know what might happen, you can make plans to deal with it. This can mean finding people who can help, learning new ways to talk to the person with dementia, or finding out what kind of medical care they will need.

It's also important to be realistic. Dementia can be different for everyone. Some people with dementia might still remember a lot, while others might forget a lot very quickly. By being realistic, you can make plans that are right for the person you're taking care of.

So, what can you do to start setting these expectations? First, learn as much as you can about dementia. There are lots of books and websites that can help you understand what it is and what to expect. You can talk to doctors and other caregivers too. They can share their experiences and the things they have learned.

Next, think about the care that the person with dementia will need. This might mean help with eating, getting dressed, or going to the doctor. Start to think about who can help with these things. It might be family, friends, or professional caregivers. Knowing who can help and how they can help is a big part of being ready. Also, think about the help that you will need. Taking care of someone with dementia can be tough. You might need a break sometimes or someone to talk to. This is okay. Remember, taking care of yourself helps you take care of others better. So, think about your own needs too.

Setting expectations for dementia care is not just about knowing the hard stuff. It's about being ready to keep loving and caring for the person with dementia, even as things change. It's about finding joy in the good moments and finding strength in the tough ones. It's about being there for them, just like you want someone to be there for you.

So, to wrap up, dementia is a tough word, but it doesn't have to be a scary one. By understanding what it is and setting the right expectations, you can make a plan that works. You can be the best caregiver you can be. And you can make sure that the person with dementia is cared for with love and respect.

Remember, you're not alone. There are lots of people and resources out there to help you on this journey. And by taking it one step at a time, you can do it. You can be a great caregiver, and you can help the person with dementia live their best life. That's what it's all about.

Acccpting Emotional Realities

When a loved one is diagnosed with dementia, it feels like a sudden storm clouding a sunny day. The news comes, and it hits hard. It's not just a word; it's a wave that washes over every part of your life. You might start to ask yourself, What does this mean? How will things change? And it's okay. It's okay to have these questions. It's more than okay to feel a whirlwind of emotions. You are human, after all.

At first, it might seem like something you can push aside. Denial is a strong force. It whispers in your ear that things are not as they seem and that the doctors might be wrong. But deep down, there's a knowing look within you. You know that pretending the problem isn't there won't make it go away. It's like covering your eyes when you're scared. Just because you can't see the thing that frightens you, it doesn't mean it's not there. The truth is that facing reality is the first step on this new path.

Guilt may creep in next. It has a tricky way of making you question everything. Did you miss the signs?

Could you have done something sooner? Listen, guilt is like a shadow that follows you around. It tries to darken every step you take. But you have to remember, you did the best with what you knew at the time. Guilt doesn't have to be the backpack you carry on this journey. You can set it down. You are doing the best you can, right here, right now. And that is enough.

Then there's grief. Grief is not just about losing someone who has passed away. It's also about saying goodbye to the future you had planned and to the way things used to be. It's a process, a long winding road with ups and downs. It might feel like you're losing your loved one bit by bit, and that's heavy. It's a burden no one should have to carry alone. But here's the thing about grief: It's also a testament to love. It shows how deep your care goes, and that's beautiful in its own way.

So how do you deal with all these feelings? You take them one at a time. You don't have to figure it all out today. You start small. Maybe today, you just acknowledge that you're feeling sad. That's a step. It's an important step.

You're recognizing what's happening in your heart. And then, maybe tomorrow, you take another step. You reach out to a friend, or you write down your thoughts in a journal. It's like walking through a fog. You can't see the end, but each step forward matters.

Strategies for dealing with these feelings are like tools in a toolbox. You have to find the right one for the job. For denial, education is key. Learn about dementia. Understand what the diagnosis really means. Knowledge is like a light in the darkness. It helps you see things more clearly. For guilt, forgiveness is your tool. Forgive yourself. Speak kindly to the person in the mirror. You're human, and humans are not perfect. And for grief, your tool is support. Lean on others. Join a support group. Share your story. You're not alone, even when it feels like it.

Remember, emotions are like the weather; they change. Some days will be sunny, and others will be stormy. That's okay. You're not alone. There are so many people walking through this storm with you. And like any weather, the storm will pass. It may not seem like it, but the sun will shine again. Until then, you carry an umbrella, you wear your rain boots, and you keep moving forward. Step by step. Together.

Think of this: Every feeling you have is a step on the path to acceptance. It's not about reaching a destination where everything is okay. It's about walking the path and knowing that every emotion is part of the journey. It's part of caring deeply for someone else. And as you walk this path, you might just find a strength you didn't know you had. That strength is what will carry you through the days ahead.

At the end of the day, the goal isn't to erase these feelings. It's to understand them and to learn how to carry them with you without letting them weigh you down. This is your journey. It's unique, hard, and sometimes lonely, but it's also filled with moments of incredible love and tenderness. And as you learn to accept these emotional realities, you start to see that love is the true heart of caregiving. It's what makes all the difference. It's what will guide you through the fog and into the light of better days.

Preparing for the Journey

When you find out you're going to be a caregiver for someone with dementia, it's like getting ready for a long trip. You know it won't be easy. You know there will be ups and downs. But just like when you pack a suitcase, there are things you can do to get ready. Let's talk about how you can prepare yourself for this important role. It's a big job, and you want to do it well. You care a lot about the person who needs your help. That's why you're here, right? To start, being a caregiver means you are there for someone else. You give them help with their day. You make sure they are safe. You show them love.

But to do this big job, you need to be strong, too. Just like when you put on your own oxygen mask before helping others on a plane, you need to take care of yourself. This is a big part of getting ready to be a caregiver. It's not just kind. It's smart.

Being balanced in your mind is key. You might feel a lot of things. You might feel sad or worried. You might even feel mad or tired sometimes. But, that's okay. Those feelings are normal. But you need to find a way to stay calm and happy, too. This will help you be the best caregiver you can be. It's not just good for you. It's good for the person you're caring for, too.

So, how do you stay balanced? First, you make time for yourself. Even if it's just a little bit each day. Maybe you love to walk, read a book, or just sit quietly. It's like charging a battery. You need to recharge so you can keep going. It's not selfish. It's smart. You are important, too. When you feel good, you can give more to others.

Then, there's your body. Taking care of your body is a big part of being ready to care for someone else. You need to eat good food, drink water, and move around. It's like giving your body the tools it needs to do a good job. Just like a car needs gas and oil to run well, your body needs good things to keep going. It's simple, but it's so important. Remember, you can't help anyone if you're sick or too tired.

Getting enough sleep is so important, too. It's like hitting a reset button for your brain. When you sleep, your body can fix things that are worn out from the day. Your mind can rest. You wake up ready to help again. So, make sure to get good sleep. It's not always easy, but it's worth it.

There's also learning. Learn all you can about dementia. Knowing what to expect can make things easier. It's like looking at a map before you go on a trip. You can see where you're going and plan the best way to get there. There are books, websites, and classes that can teach you about dementia. You can learn about what the person you're caring for might do or feel. This can help you understand them better. It can help you be patient. It can help you make good choices for their care.

Remember, you're not alone! So many people are caring for someone with dementia. They know what you're going through. They can give you tips or just listen when you need to talk. They can help you remember that you're doing a great job. Sometimes, just knowing someone else understands can make a big difference.

And remember to laugh. Yes, laugh! Laughter is like sunshine for your heart. It makes you feel light and happy. It chases away the dark thoughts. Find things that make you laugh. A funny movie, a joke, a silly dance. It doesn't matter what it is. Laughter is good medicine. It can keep you going on tough days. You also need to plan. Plan for what you need to do each day. Plan for what might happen in the future. It's like packing your bag. You think about what you will need. Then, you make sure you have it. This could mean making lists or setting up a schedule. It could mean talking to doctors or looking for helpers. It means thinking ahead. This way, when things change, you're ready for them.

Finally, take one day at a time. You can't do everything at once. It's like climbing a mountain. You can't jump to the top. You take one step at a time. Do what you can each day. Some days will be hard. Some days will be easier. But each day, you're doing something amazing. You're caring for someone who needs you. That's a beautiful thing.

So, let's get ready for this journey. It's a big one, but you can do it. You're strong. You're caring. And you have a big heart. That's the best tool of all. Now, go ahead. Take that first step. Take care of yourself. Learn. Plan. Laugh. And remember, you're not alone. We're here with you. Step by step, day by day, you'll make this journey. And it will make all the difference in the world to the person you love.

Building a Support System

When you're caring for someone with dementia, having people around who understand what you're going through is like having a net below a tightrope. It's there to catch you if you slip. This is why building a support system is so vital. A support system isn't just a group of people. It's your own personal team. This team can help you through the tough days and celebrate the good ones with you.

Let's talk about where to start. Finding resources and communities can seem big and confusing, but it's actually simple when you break it down. You want to look for people and places that give you strength and guidance. This could be a support group, a healthcare professional, or other caregivers. They're out there, and they're ready to help you. You just need to reach out.

Support groups are like having a friend who knows exactly what you're dealing with. They're made up of people just like you. People who are caring for someone with dementia. They meet up, either in person or online.

At these meetings, they share their stories. They talk about what's hard. They share what works for them. And they listen to you when you need to talk. In a support group, you'll find shoulders to lean on and hands to hold. They'll give you advice that's worked for them, which might work for you, too.

Next, healthcare professionals are like guides in the confusing world of dementia care. They know a lot about the disease. They can tell you what to expect and how to handle different situations. You can find these professionals at clinics and hospitals. They can answer your questions, give you advice, and connect you with other resources. Talking to them can make a big difference in how you care for your loved one. Then there are other caregivers. They're in the same boat as you. Some may have been doing this for a long time. Others might be new, just like you. They all have experiences and ideas that can help you. You can meet them in support groups, at clinics, or even in online forums. When you share with them and they share with you, it's like trading tools to make your job easier. They understand the ups and downs because they're living them, too.

Connecting with these resources and communities starts with a phone call or a click on the internet. It's as simple as searching for "dementia support groups near me" or asking your doctor for recommendations. And remember, joining these groups or talking to these people doesn't mean you can't handle your situation. It means you're smart. You're gathering all the tools and all the friends you can to help you care for your loved one.

So, reach out. Start building your support system today. It's one of the most important things you can do as a caregiver. With this support system, you'll find comfort, advice, and maybe even some new friends. And when things get tough, you'll have a whole team behind you, ready to help you stand up again. Remember, you're not alone on this journey. And with the right support system, you'll find the strength you need to face each day with hope and love.

Establishing a Care Framework

Caregiving is a journey that requires patience, understanding, and a well-thought-out plan. When someone we love receives a dementia diagnosis, we step into a role that is both new and challenging. Establishing a care framework is about laying a foundation that can support the shifting landscape of needs that come with dementia. This involves crafting routines and strategies that are flexible and responsive to these changes.

First, let's talk about what a care framework really means. It's like a map for your caregiving journey. Now, a map helps you know where you're going, what turns to take, and when to stop for rest. Just like that, a care framework guides you in providing the best care possible. It's not just a daily plan; it's an approach that evolves and adapts over time.

Creating this framework starts with understanding the person you're caring for. Their likes, dislikes, habits, and routines. This is vital. You want to maintain a sense of normalcy and comfort for them. So, take the time to really think about what makes them happy. Maybe it's a morning walk, a specific meal they enjoy, or a favorite song. These details might seem small, but they make a huge difference.

Next, consider the tasks that need to be accomplished each day. Things like medication management, doctor's appointments, meals, and personal care. Write these down. By listing them, you create a visual reminder of what needs to be done. It also helps you to organize these tasks in a way that flows naturally with your loved one's best times of day. Maybe mornings are good for them; maybe afternoons are better.

Let's not forget about flexibility. Dementia can change how a person feels from one day to the next, or even from one hour to the next. Your care framework must have room for these changes. If your loved one is having a bad day, it's okay to shift things around. The point is always to focus on what is best for them at that moment.

Now, routines are important. They bring stability and predictability, which can be comforting for someone with dementia. So, try to keep meal times, bedtimes, and other activities as regular as possible. But remember, it's okay if things don't always go as planned. Be gentle with yourself and your loved ones. It's the love and care you give that matter most, not sticking to a strict schedule.

One more thing to consider is communication. With dementia, communication can become difficult. It's essential to learn ways to connect without causing frustration. Simple words, a calm voice, and even non-verbal cues like smiling can speak volumes. Always approach your loved one with a gentle presence. This helps them feel safe and understood.

As you put your care framework into action, remember to take care of yourself too. Caregiving is a demanding job, and you need to be in good shape to do it well. Make sure to schedule time for yourself, even if it's just a few minutes to breathe and relax. Your well-being is just as important as the care you provide.

Finally, the care framework isn't set in stone. It's a living document of sorts. You'll adjust it as you learn more about what works and what doesn't. Keep notes on what you notice each day. These notes will be invaluable as you fine-tune your approach.

So, what do you walk away with from all of this? You have a clearer idea of what it means to establish a care framework. You understand the importance of knowing the person you care for and maintaining routines while also staying flexible. You've learned that communication is key and that your own health should never be put on the back burner. All of this knits together into a strategy that respects both your loved one's needs and your capacity to meet them.

Now, take these ideas and start to apply them. Look at your caregiving situation through this lens of adaptable structure. Begin by mapping out a simple routine for tomorrow. Use what you've learned here to make each caregiving day a little better than the last. And remember, you're not alone on this journey. There's a community of caregivers out there, all learning and growing together. You're a part of that now, and together, we can make each step forward a meaningful one.

Recap: The Path Ahead

So far, we've taken quite the journey together. We've looked into what dementia is and how it can change lives. We've talked about the feelings you might have when someone you care for gets this diagnosis. There's a lot to handle, but remember, you're not alone. Let's take a moment to breathe and think about what we've learned.

We started by setting the stage for what dementia care involves. It's a big task, but knowing what to expect makes it easier. You learned that it's okay to feel all sorts of emotions. You might feel sad, confused, or even angry. That's normal. You're human, after all.

Then, we moved on to getting ready for what's ahead. It's like packing for a trip. You want to make sure you have everything you need. Preparing isn't just about having the right supplies. It's also about making sure you're ready inside your mind and your heart.

We also talked about people who can help. Like finding a team for a big project, you want to have good people around you. There are groups you can join, professionals who understand, and folks just like you. They're all part of your team now.

And we can't forget about making a plan. It's like building a house. You need a good foundation and a strong frame so it can last a long time. Your care plan needs to be strong too. It will change over time, but starting with something solid is key.

Here are some steps to take right now:

Write down your thoughts and feelings. This can help clear your head and make things less scary.

- Make a list of questions you have about dementia. You can take this to a doctor or a support group.

- Look for a caregiver group you can join. It's good to talk to people who understand what you're going through.

- Set aside some time every day just for you. You need to take care of yourself to take care of someone else.

- Start making a daily plan for your loved one with dementia. Think about meals, rest, and fun activities.

- Learn one new thing about dementia this week. Understanding more can make you feel more in control.

- Talk to a friend or family member about your caregiving. It's okay to ask for help when you need it.

- Think about the future and write down what you hope for. This can give you something positive to focus on.

Remember, you're learning to be a great caregiver. It's a big job, but you can do it. You have a heart full of love and hands ready to help. Your loved one is lucky to have you. And you're not alone. There are so many resources and people ready to stand with you. Take a deep breath. You're stepping onto a path that many have walked before.

Each step might feel heavy sometimes, but you have the strength to move forward. And as you walk this path, you'll find that you're able to do more than you ever thought possible.

As we close this chapter, think about the journey ahead with hope. You've got the tools, the support, and the plan to make it through. You're ready to be the best caregiver you can be. And that's a beautiful thing. Keep these steps close to your heart, and when you're feeling lost, look back at them. They're your guide on this path. One step at a time, one day at a time.

And if you ever need a reminder of why you're doing this, just look into the eyes of the person you're caring for. You'll see the love and trust there. That's what makes it all worth it. That's what keeps you going. You're doing something amazing, and I'm here cheering you on every step of the way.

So, stay strong, be kind to yourself, and embrace the journey. You're not just a caregiver; you're a hero in someone's story. And that's something truly special. Ready? Let's keep moving forward together.

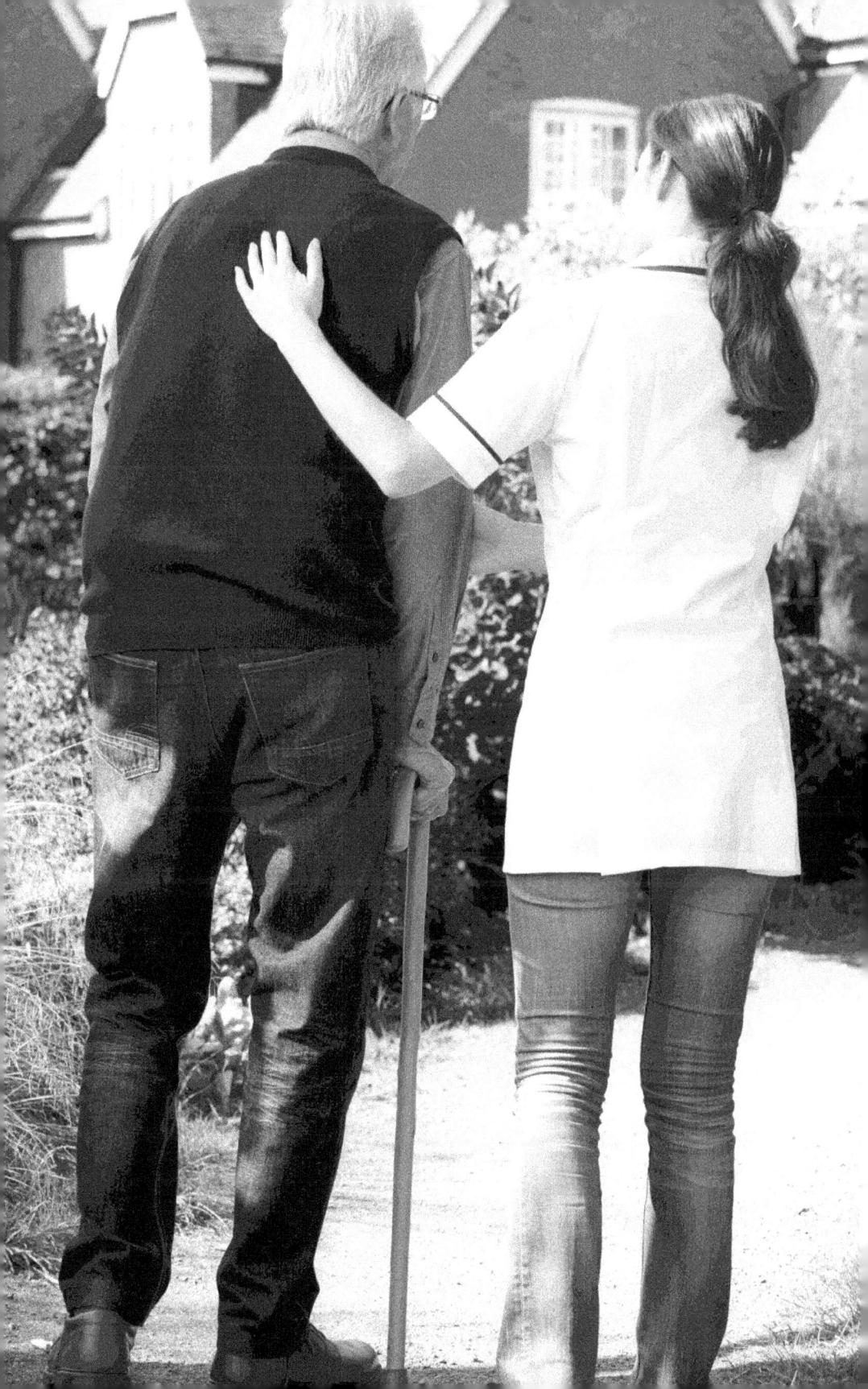

Chapter Three.
Mindfulness in Caregiving

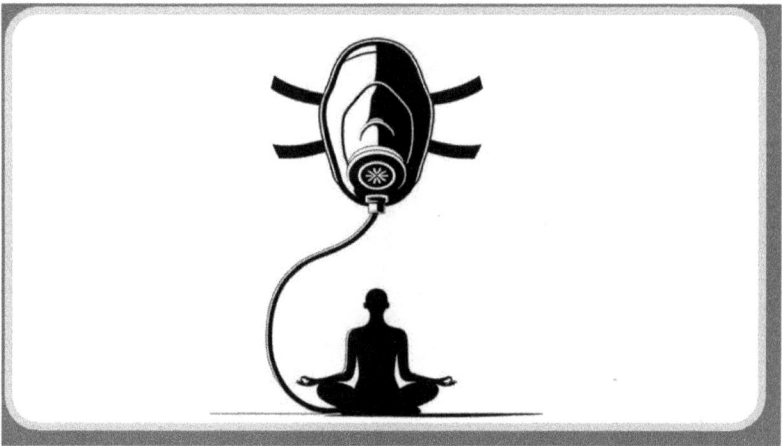

"Like airplane passengers, let's not forget to put our own oxygen masks first…we are no good to our loved ones if we collapse under the strain."

– Peter B

The Role of Mindfulness

The idea of mindfulness might seem like a big word. We hear it a lot these days. But what does it actually mean, especially when we talk about taking care of someone else?

Mindfulness is really about being fully there. When you're with someone, you're really with them— not just in the same room, but with your mind too. You're not thinking about the grocery list or the TV show you watched last night. It's about being present in the moment.

So, why is this important for someone who is caring for another person? Think of it this way: When you're truly there, you can see what the person you're taking care of needs right away. You can hear the little things in their voice that tell you how they're feeling. It's like turning up the volume on your attention. And for someone with dementia, having someone pay that kind of close attention can make a big difference. It can make them feel safe and understood.

But mindfulness isn't just about being there for someone else. It's also for you, the caregiver. When you practice being mindful, you might notice that you start to feel less stressed. That's a big deal because stress can make you feel tired and make it hard to think. It can even make you sick. But when you're mindful, you take a step back. You breathe. You notice the stress but don't let it take over.

Being a caregiver is tough. It asks a lot of you. When you're mindful, you give yourself a break. You find little moments of quiet in your day. These moments help you recharge. They're like a little rest stop on a long trip. And when you have that rest, you can give more to the person you take care of. You have more patience, and more kindness. Your smile comes easier—all because you took a moment to just be.

Now, how do you do it?

How do you become mindful when you're busy and have so much to think about? The good news is that it's simple. You don't need special things to get started.

It's as easy as taking a deep breath. As you breathe out, think about letting go of your worries—just for that breath. And then do it again and again. Each breath is a step towards being more mindful.

You might think, "Can something so simple really make a difference?" The answer is yes, it can. When you do this breathing exercise, you might start to notice other things—like the way the air feels cool going into your nose and warm coming out, or the way your chest rises and falls. You're starting to pay attention to the little things. That's mindfulness. And when you do that during the day, you bring that attention with you as you take care of someone.

This isn't a race. You don't need to be perfect at being mindful right away. It takes practice, like learning to play an instrument or riding a bike. But each time you do it, you get better. You start to feel the benefits, and that's a good reason to keep at it.

Mindfulness isn't just another task on your to-do list. It's a new way to see your day and your job as a caregiver. It's a way to make everything a bit calmer and brighter for you and for the person you care for. And that's something worth trying, don't you think?

Mindfulness Techniques

Mindfulness is like a gentle wave that washes over our busy lives. It's a practice that asks us to slow down, to breathe, and to be in this single moment. For caregivers, it's a breath of fresh air in a room that sometimes feels too stuffy or busy. It's important to learn mindfulness techniques because they can bring calm to our days and help us care for others with a kind heart.

Now, mindfulness isn't complex. It's about being right here, right now, with all of your focus. It's like when you listen to your favorite song, and nothing else matters—that's being mindful. Let's walk through some basic practices that you can use every day to bring you into the present moment.

First, there's breathing. Sit down. Close your eyes. Now, take a deep breath. Feel your chest and belly rise. Hold it. Let it out slowly. Feel the air leave your body. This is mindful breathing. It's easy but powerful. Do this a few times, and it will help calm your mind. You can do this anytime, anywhere, when you feel stressed or rushed.

Another technique is called body scanning. Lie down or sit comfortably. Close your eyes. Think about your toes. How do they feel? Are they warm or cold, tense or relaxed? Slowly move your mind up your body, from toes to head. Notice every part. If you find tense spots, breathe into them. Imagine the tension melting away. This scan isn't quick; it's slow and careful. It connects you to your body and eases tension.

Using Mindfulness When Things Get Tough

Caregiving isn't easy. It can be really stressful, but mindfulness can help you even in the hardest times. Say you're helping someone who is upset. You feel your heart beat faster, and stress rises. Now is the time to be mindful. Focus on your breathing. In, out. Stay calm. This helps both you and the person you're caring for. You become a calm spot in a stormy sea—that's how powerful mindfulness can be.

These techniques can be part of your day like breakfast is part of your morning. Work them into your routine. Maybe you start with breathing when you wake up, then do a body scan at lunch. When you feel stressed, focus on your breath. It doesn't need to be a big thing. It's a small thing with a big effect. Like drops of water filling a cup, little by little, your mindfulness practice grows.

Integrating Mindfulness with Care

When we speak of integrating mindfulness with care, particularly in the scope of caring for individuals with dementia, we are talking about a very focused way of being. This requires us to be present, patient, and compassionate in every interaction. Let's dive into what this entails and how to make it a reality in your daily care routine.

Mindful Communication

Mindful communication means that when you talk to someone with dementia, you give them your full attention. You listen to their words, tone, and body language. You do this because it helps you understand what they need and feel.

This is not just about being a good listener—it's about connecting with the person on a deeper level. Imagine you're having a conversation. If your mind is full of other thoughts, you might miss something important. But when you're mindful, you catch every detail. It's like tuning into a radio frequency where the signal is clear without any static. You're not just hearing words—you're feeling emotions and sensing needs.

So, how do you practice mindful communication? It starts with silence. Before you even begin talking, take a moment to clear your mind. Take a deep breath and let go of other thoughts. Look at the person you're caring for and see them as they are right now. When they speak, focus solely on their words and respond with care and thoughtfulness. If they're upset, your calm presence can help soothe them. If they're happy, your shared attention can amplify their joy.

Mindful Observation

When words fail, this is where mindful observation comes in. With dementia patients, sometimes their actions and behaviors tell you more than words ever could. This means watching with a keen eye, and noticing the little things.

For instance, if the person you care for is fidgeting or looks uncomfortable, they may be in pain but unable to express it. If they avoid eye contact, they might feel overwhelmed or scared. By observing these signs, you can adjust your care to meet their needs without them having to tell you.

To practice mindful observation, you need to slow down. When you're helping them eat, don't rush. Watch how they handle their utensils. Are they struggling? Are they disinterested in food? These observations can guide you in making mealtime more comfortable and enjoyable for them.

Mindfulness for Self-Care

When we talk about caregiving, a picture forms in our minds. It's one of giving, supporting, and doing for others. Yet, today, we're turning the lens around. Let's look at the caregiver. If that's you, it's time we focus on your well-being. How, you ask? Through the power of mindfulness.

Why is self-care crucial for you as a caregiver? Think of it like this: if you have a cup full of water, you can give others a drink. But if your cup is empty, you have nothing to offer. Your well-being is that cup. Mindfulness is a way to keep it full. It's about being in the moment, aware, and fully present. And it's not just good for the mind—it's food for the soul too.

Now, let's talk about creating a routine. You might say, "But I'm so busy already!" Sure, caregiving can fill up a schedule. Yet, remember that cup we talked about? It needs refilling. And that means making time. Here's the good news: mindfulness doesn't take hours. Just a few moments can make a real difference. Start in the morning. Can you spare five minutes? Sit in a quiet spot. Close your eyes. Take deep breaths. Inhale. Exhale. Feel the air moving in and out. Notice how the chair holds you, how your feet touch the floor. This is you, being in the now. This is mindfulness.

But what about those times when stress bubbles up? When the person you care for is having a tough day? That's when mindfulness can be a superhero. A quick pause. A few deep breaths. Remind yourself: "I'm here. I'm okay." It's like hitting the reset button for your brain. And guess what? You'll be calmer. That calm can spread to the person you're caring for.

Maybe you're saying, "This sounds nice, but I'll forget to do it." That's okay. It's normal. What can help? Reminders. Sticky notes on the mirror. An alarm on your phone. A note in your pocket. Little nudges to bring you back to mindfulness. Each time you remember, that's a win. That's you, taking care of your cup.

Here's a secret: mindfulness isn't just sitting still. It's in the little things. Washing dishes? Feel the water.

Hear the clink of dishes. Walking? Notice your steps, the air on your face. Each moment is a chance to practice, to be aware, to fill your cup. And as you keep at it, something amazing happens. You'll notice changes. Maybe you're not as quick to worry. Maybe you smile more. Maybe you find joy in small things. That's the power of a regular mindfulness routine. It's like watering a plant. Be consistent, and it will grow.

So, what's your takeaway? Mindfulness is your tool, your self-care kit. It's there for you, in the quiet mornings and the busy afternoons. Use it to keep yourself well. Because when you're well, you can give so much more. And that's not just good for you—it's a gift to those you care for.

If you ever feel lost, remember this: just breathe. Just be. The rest will follow. And if you need a friend to guide you, we're here. Join our community, and subscribe to our newsletter. We've got courses, resources, and a listening ear. We believe in caring for the caregiver, and we can't wait to welcome you.

Mindfulness in Practice

Now, it's important to acknowledge that learning to integrate mindfulness with care takes practice. It doesn't happen overnight. But every small step you take is progress. Each time you communicate mindfully or observe with compassion, you're building a stronger, more patient, and understanding relationship with the person you're caring for.

So, start small. Pick one aspect of your caregiving routine—perhaps mealtimes or getting dressed—and focus on being completely present. Notice the difference it makes, not just for the person you're caring for but for you as well. It can transform the experience from a task into a meaningful interaction.

SCAN THIS AND LEARN MORE ABOUT
CAREGIVERS TODAY

When you join a community, you can connect with other caregivers and get the support you need on this journey. This is not just about providing care; it's about caring with intention, focus, and heart. And we're here to do it together. So, take these lessons and integrate them into your caregiving. Use them to change your approach, improve your methods, and ultimately enhance the lives of those you care for. It's a powerful step towards compassionate care, and it starts with mindfulness.

Overcoming Barriers to Mindfulness

Mindfulness is a simple practice, but don't let its simplicity fool you. It's powerful, and it can change how you act as a caregiver. Yet, it's not always easy. You might find it hard to be mindful. You might try and feel like it's not working. That's normal. Let's talk about these barriers and how to stick with them, even when it's tough.

First, what stops us from being mindful? You might be too busy. You have a lot to do, and it's hard to find time to stop and just be in the moment. Or maybe you feel like you can't do it right. That's a common thought. Here's what you should know: being mindful isn't about being perfect. It's about trying. It's about doing it again and again. It's about coming back to the moment whenever you can.

Another barrier is feeling like it's not working. You might sit still and close your eyes, trying to focus on your breathing, but your mind is full of thoughts. You're thinking about what you need to do, worrying about the person you're caring for. It feels like you're failing at being mindful. But guess what? Noticing that your mind has wandered is an act of mindfulness. Each time you bring your focus back, you're succeeding. It's like lifting weights—it makes you stronger every time you do it.

How to Keep Going

So, how do you keep going? How do you make sure you keep being mindful? It's about making it a habit. It's about finding a little bit of time each day. Maybe it's just a few minutes in the morning, or while you're washing dishes. You can be mindful anytime, anywhere. It's flexible.

Staying committed to practice is key. How? One way is to remember why you're doing it. Think about the calm it can bring you. Think about how it can help you take better care of your loved one. Keep those benefits in mind—they can motivate you to keep going.

Another way is to set small goals. Say to yourself, "I'll be mindful for one minute today." When that feels easy, make it two minutes. Gradually, your mindfulness muscle grows. Before you know it, being mindful is a normal part of your day.

It also helps to have reminders. Put a sticky note on your fridge. It could say, "Take a deep breath." Have an alarm on your phone that says, "Pause. Feel your feet on the ground." These little cues can bring you back to the present moment. They can help you weave mindfulness into your day.

And it's okay to ask for help. Maybe you can join a group. There are groups for caregivers who understand what you're going through. They can support you and remind you to be mindful. You're not alone. Together, you can keep the practice of mindfulness alive.

Let's not forget the simple acts that can help. Maybe you take a walk. Notice the air on your skin. Listen to the birds. Feel each step you take. These are moments of mindfulness. They can refresh you. They can make a difference in your day.

Remember, it's not about how long you're mindful—it's about the quality. It's about truly being where you are. Even a few seconds can change your mood. It can change how you talk to the person you're caring for. It can change the care you give. Mindfulness is a gift to yourself and the person you care for. Every effort you make counts. Each moment of mindfulness adds up. It makes life a little brighter. It makes caregiving a little lighter. And it makes your heart a little fuller. So, take a deep breath right now. Feel it. Be here. You're doing great. Just keep going, one breath at a time.

Recap: Being Present

Caregiving is a role that comes with many challenges. It's easy to get caught up in the never-ending list of tasks. There's always something that needs to be done, right? While you're ticking off those tasks, it can be hard to stay focused on the present moment. This is where mindfulness comes into play. It's like a gentle hand on your shoulder, reminding you to slow down and be here right now. That's what we've been discussing, and it's essential.

You see, mindfulness is not just about being calm. It's about being awake to the life you are living at this very moment. It's about noticing the colors, smells, and sounds around you. It's about really seeing the person you're caring for, listening to them, and understanding them. Being present means not thinking about what you'll have for dinner while helping someone else with their meal. It means not planning your next task while you're still doing the current one.

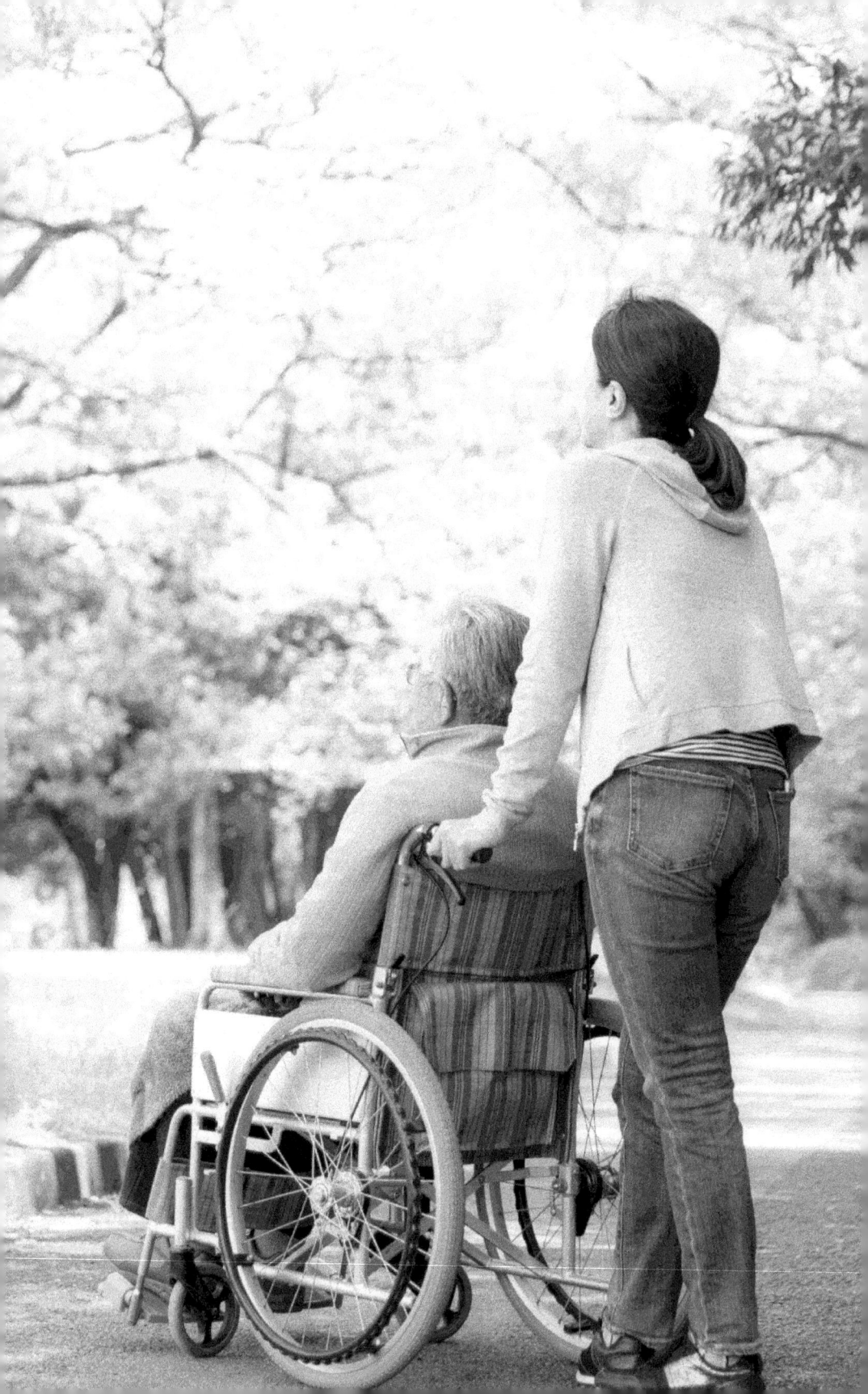

Chapter Four.
Patience with Progress

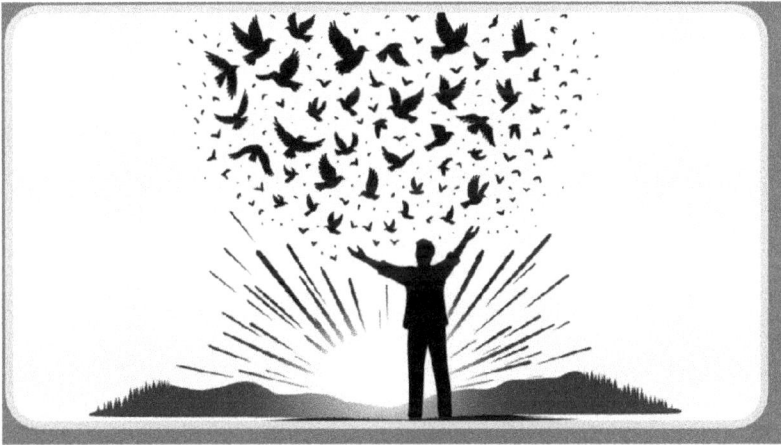

"Caring about others, running the risk of feeling, and leaving an impact on people, bring happiness."

– Harold Kushner

Patience is like a quiet friend who helps us through tough times. In the world of caring for someone with dementia, patience isn't just helpful; it's a must-have. You see, when someone you care for has dementia, things can change a lot. Some days might be good, and some days might be hard. But with patience, you can make each day a bit better for both of you.

Now, let's talk about why patience is so important. When you're patient, you give the person with dementia the space they need. They might take longer to do things or remember stuff. But when you're patient, you tell them it's okay. You tell them they can take their time and that you're there with them every step of the way. But how do you stay patient, especially on tough days? That's where setting realistic expectations comes in. This means understanding that things might not go as quickly as you'd like. It's all about taking a deep breath and remembering that progress, no matter how small, is still progress.

Let's dive deeper into setting those expectations. It's important to know that each day with dementia can be different. Some days, the person you care for might remember your name, and other days, they might not. This can feel hard, but it's part of the journey. When you expect that each day can be different, it helps you stay calm and patient. Now, think about the small things. Maybe today, the person you care for was able to eat their breakfast without help. That's a victory! It's a sign of progress, and it's something to be happy about. Celebrating these small wins helps you see the good in every day, and it keeps your patience strong.

Imagine you're walking on a long road with no end in sight. That's what it can feel like when you're caring for someone with dementia. But if you look down at your feet, you'll see you're actually taking steps forward. That's what progress in dementia care is like. It might feel slow, but with patience, you'll see that you're moving forward, one step at a time.

What about those days when you feel like you can't be patient anymore? It's normal to feel that way sometimes. The trick is to have some tools to help you find your patience again. One tool is to take breaks. Yes, it's okay to step away for a moment and just breathe. Maybe you can take a walk or listen to your favorite song. It's not just okay; it's important. It helps you come back refreshed and ready to be patient again. Another tool is talking to friends or joining a group of caregivers. These people understand what you're going through. They can give you support and share their tips for being patient. Plus, it feels good to talk about your day and hear that others have tough days too. It reminds you that you're not alone. Being patient doesn't mean you're perfect. It just means you're trying your best. And that's all anyone can ask for. So, take it one day at a time. Be kind to yourself and to the person you care for. And remember, patience is your friend on this journey. It's there to help you through the slow times and the tough times. With patience, you can do this. You can care for your loved one with dementia and do it with love and kindness.

And that's the heart of it, isn't it? It's all about love. Being patient is a way of showing love. It says, "I'm here for you, no matter what." That's a powerful message. So, embrace patience. Let it be your guide. Know that, with patience, you're giving the very best care you can. That's something to be proud of.

Before we wrap up, let's think about what you can do today to be more patient. Maybe you can write down one small goal for the day. Something simple, like helping your loved one with a puzzle or just sitting with them and listening to music, and at the end of the day, look back at that goal. If you reached it, great! If not, that's okay too. Just trying is a step forward. And each step forward is a reason to celebrate.

So, as you move through your day, hold onto patience. Keep it close, and let it guide you. With patience, you'll find the strength you didn't know you had. And you'll see that even on the hardest days, there's always a reason to hope. Because with each little step, you're making life a bit better for the person you love. And that's what caregiving is all about.

Remember, patience isn't just a nice thing to have. It's the key to being a great caregiver. So, take a deep breath, set realistic expectations, and let patience lead the way. And when you do, you'll find that you're not just getting through the days; you're making them count. You're making a difference. And that's what truly matters.

Thanks for taking this time to think about patience in dementia care. It's a big topic, but you've got this. You have the tools, the support, and the love to make each day a good one. So, keep going, keep caring, and keep being the amazing caregiver you are. Your loved one is lucky to have you. And remember, we're here for you every step of the way.

Managing Expectations

When caring for someone with dementia, we all hope to see signs of improvement, big or small. Yet, real progress can be slow. Very slow. At times, it is like watching a flower bloom in slow motion. You know it's happening, but it's happening at its own pace, a pace we cannot rush.

Now, let's talk about expectations. Expectations are what we think should happen. We might expect a person with dementia to remember what we told them yesterday. Or we might expect them to learn a new daily routine after a couple of tries. But the truth is, that dementia works differently. And that means we need to change our expectations to fit this new reality.

But why are expectations so important? If we set the bar too high, we set ourselves up for disappointment. We feel sad when things don't go as planned. On the other side, if we expect too little, we might not try enough. So, what we need is a balance. A way to hope for the best but still be okay when things go slow.

To do this, we need techniques. Techniques are like tools. They help us do our jobs better. They can help us set these realistic expectations. One technique is to make small goals. Not big ones, just tiny steps. Think about teaching a child to put on their shoes. You don't start with laces. You start by just putting a foot in. And celebrate that. It's the same with dementia care.

Another technique is to write things down. When we write down what happens each day, we can see progress over time. It's easy to forget small changes. But when they're on paper, we can look back and see them clearly. It's like leaving a trail of breadcrumbs. They show us where we've been and how far we've come.

Now, acknowledging small victories is a big deal. Imagine a day when the person you care for remembers your name. It might not happen every day, but when it does, it's a win. It's a moment to hold on to. A small victory. We collect these moments like precious stones. Each one is a treasure.

Some days might be hard. You might feel like there's been no progress at all. But this is where our techniques come in. We look at our notes. We remember the small victories. And we remind ourselves that slow progress is still progress. We're on a journey that doesn't have a map. We make our own map as we go along.

To manage expectations, we have to be patient. Patience is like a warm blanket on a cold day. It comforts us. It reminds us that it's okay to move slowly. It tells us that we're doing just fine, even when things don't seem fine.

Patience is our friend in the world of dementia care. We also need to tell our hearts to be patient too. Our hearts want everything to be okay right now. But our minds know that's not how it works. So we gently tell our hearts to wait. To trust that we're doing our best. And our best is good enough.

In a way, managing expectations is like growing a garden. We plant seeds. We water them. We give them sunlight. But we cannot make them grow faster than they want to. They will sprout in their own time. And when they do, it's a beautiful sight.

So, let's be gardeners of patience. Let's set realistic goals. Let's write our notes. Let's celebrate every tiny victory. Let's be patient with our hearts. And let's keep going, even on the slow days. Because every step forward, no matter how small, is a step in the right direction.

Remember, this journey is not a race. There's no finish line to rush to. It's a walk through a path we're making. We're walking it together, with the person we care for. We're learning, growing, and finding joy in the little things. And that's what matters.

Let's wrap this up with something you can do right now. Pick a small goal for the week. It could be anything. Maybe it's getting a smile from the person you care for. Or maybe it's just having a peaceful meal together. Write it down. And at the end of the week, check-in.

Did you reach your goal? If you did, celebrate! If not, it's okay. Learn from it. And set a new goal for next week. This way, you're taking steps. You're moving forward. And you're doing it with love, patience, and realistic expectations.

Patience in Communication

Caregiving is a journey. On this journey, one of the most precious things you can carry with you is patience. Now, let's talk about patience when you're talking with someone who has dementia. It's a special kind of patience. It's not just waiting quietly. It's about how you make them feel heard and understood. When you talk to someone with dementia, it might seem hard at first. They might forget what they were saying, or they might say things that don't make sense to you. But with the right way of speaking and listening, you can make a big difference.

First, you need to know that taking your time is okay. When they are trying to find the right words, give them space. Don't rush them. If they are slow to answer, wait a bit. They are doing their best, and so are you. Smiling helps a lot. It makes them feel safe and happy. Even if they forget your words, they won't forget how you made them feel.

Next, let's think about how you talk. Use simple words. Big, fancy words can be confusing. Talk about one thing at a time. This helps them understand better. If you're talking about going to the park, just talk about the park. Don't talk about the park, the weather, and what you'll eat for lunch all at once. Break it down. One thing at a time.

Sometimes, they might get upset or angry. This is normal. Remember, it's not about you. They're dealing with a lot in their own minds. Stay calm. Use a gentle voice. If they are scared or confused, your calm voice can be like a soft blanket on a cold night. It can make them feel better.

When you listen, really listen. Look them in the eyes. Nod your head. This shows them you are with them. You care. And if they repeat themselves, it's okay. Just listen again. They need to know you're there, even if they say the same thing ten times. You can also use pictures or other things they like to help them talk. If they love cats, maybe have a picture of a cat with you. This can help them talk about what they like. It can make talking easier and more fun for them. And for you, too!

Here's something else you can do. Write down important things. If you're planning to go somewhere or do something special, write it on paper. Put the paper where they can see it. This can help remind them. It's like leaving little signposts along the path of your day together. It makes the journey smoother.

Now, all this patience in talking is not just for them. It's for you too. When you have patience, you feel better. You don't get as tired or as upset. You can be a better caregiver and enjoy your time with them more. So, when you talk to them, think of it like watering a plant. You're showing kindness and patience, and in time, you'll see them bloom a little more each day.

Lastly, let's remember that it's not about being perfect. It's about trying your best. Some days will be harder. That's life. But every day you try, you're doing something beautiful. You're giving someone the gift of patience and understanding. That's something really special. So, every day, take a deep breath. Smile. Talk gently, listen well, and know that you're doing an amazing thing.

Cultivating Patience in Daily Routines

When we care for someone with dementia, each day brings new challenges. It's like every morning starts a new adventure. Some days, we might get a smile or a thank you. On other days, we might face confusion or sadness. These ups and downs are normal. They are part of the journey. And this journey needs something very special from us. It needs patience.

Patience isn't just waiting. It's not just sitting back and hoping things will get better. No. Patience is active. It's a skill. And like any skill, it can be learned and improved. To have patience is to understand time. To know that some things can't be rushed. And in the world of caregiving, where every little task can feel like a mountain, patience becomes your best friend.

But how do we make patience part of our daily routine? It starts with the little things. It starts the moment you wake up. You take a deep breath. You feel the air fill your lungs. Then, you let it out slowly. This is your first act of patience for the day. And it's important. Because it sets the tone for everything that follows.

Next, you think about the day ahead. You make a plan. You know that the plan might change. And that's okay. The plan is a guide, not a rule. Because in dementia care, every day is different. We can't control everything. But we can control how we react. We can choose to stay calm. To be patient. And this choice? It's powerful.

As you start the day's tasks, remember to take your time. Let's say you're helping your loved one get dressed. They might be moving slowly. They might be confused. This is a moment for patience. Talk to them gently. Guide their arms through the sleeves. If they resist, don't push. Don't rush. Pause. Breathe. Try again. Or take a break and come back to it later.

During meals, patience is key too. Eating can be hard for someone with dementia. They might forget how to use a fork. They might not feel hungry. This is when you need to be patient. You can encourage them. You might say, "Here's your favorite food." You might help guide the fork to their mouth. But if they're not ready, you wait. You give them space. You can try again later.

There will be tough times. Times when you feel like you're at the end of your rope. Maybe your loved one is upset. Maybe they're repeating the same question over and over. In these moments, patience is a gift you give to both of you. You listen to the question. You answer it again and again as if it's the first time. And you do it with love. Because that's what patience is. It's love in action.

It's also important to take care of yourself. To be patient, you need to be strong. And to be strong, you need rest. So make sure you find time for yourself. Even if it's just a few minutes. Take a walk. Read a book. Sit in the garden. Do something that makes you happy. Because when you're happy, you can be more patient. And when you're patient, you're a better caregiver.

Finally, as the day comes to a close, reflect on everything that happened. Think about the good moments. The smile you shared. The laugh you had. And think about the hard parts. The times you felt like you couldn't do it. But you did. You made it through another day. And that's something to be proud of. Because it takes a special person to do what you do. It takes patience. And you have it. You've been practicing it all day.

So, as we wrap up this talk, remember that patience isn't just a feeling. It's an action. It's something you do. And the more you practice, the better you get. Tomorrow is another day. Another chance to be patient. And you're ready. You've got this.

And remember, our community is about supporting each other. About growing together. So, as you continue on this journey, know that we're with you. Every step. Every day. With patience, with love, and with care.

Overcoming Impatience and Frustration

It happens. You are caring for someone with dementia, and you feel the heat rising. Not the kind of warmth that comes from a hug or a cozy blanket, but the heat of impatience, and frustration bubbling up inside you. It's a natural feeling, but you know it doesn't help. So, what do you do? You learn to cope and manage these feelings so you can get back to providing the loving, patient care your loved one needs. Let's talk about how.

First off, know that feeling impatient or frustrated does not mean you are doing a bad job. It simply means you are human. Caring for someone with dementia is a marathon, not a sprint. It's okay to feel overwhelmed at times. What's important is how you handle these feelings. Recognizing when you are starting to feel impatient is the first step in overcoming it. Once you recognize that you're feeling impatient, take a deep breath. Breathing deeply helps calm your body and mind.

It's like when you blow up a balloon too fast, it pops. But if you blow it up slowly, it grows big and strong. Your patience works the same way. Give it time and care, and it will be stronger.

Sometimes, taking a short break can work wonders. Step out of the room for a moment, have a glass of water, walk around the garden, or just sit quietly. It's like hitting the pause button on a movie. You're not stopping the movie, just taking a brief break so you can enjoy the rest of it more. It's also helpful to remind yourself of the goal. The goal is not to rush through tasks, but to provide care with love and patience. It's not about how quickly you can complete a task, but how well you can do it while keeping the atmosphere calm and supportive. You want to be like a gentle stream, not a rushing river.

Now, let's talk about self-regulation. Self-regulation is like being the boss of your feelings. It means you decide how to react to things. If you feel impatient, tell yourself to take it easy. Remind yourself that you are in control, not your feelings. You can choose patience. Maintaining a positive outlook is key. Think about the good moments with your loved one. Maybe it's a smile, a word, or just a peaceful moment together. These good memories are like sunshine on a cloudy day. They can brighten up the toughest moments and remind you why you're doing this. Remember, you're not alone. Talk to friends, family, or a support group. These people are like your personal cheerleaders. They can lift you up, offer advice, and remind you that what you're doing is amazing. Sharing your struggles can help lighten the load.

Lastly, let's talk about planning ahead. When you have a plan, you're like a captain steering a ship through calm waters. Make a plan for those tough moments. Have activities that calm you and get you ready to go. It could be music, exercise, or reading. Then, when you feel the waves of impatience, you have your tools ready to navigate back to calm seas.

Being patient is not about being perfect. It's about trying your best every day. And when you hit bumps in the road, you deal with them calmly and carry on. Your journey of caregiving is important, and with these strategies in your toolbox, you'll be prepared to face the challenges with a steady hand and a caring heart.

So, take this advice and use it. Next time you feel impatience coming on, remember to breathe, take a break, and focus on the positive. With these simple, actionable steps, you'll find your way back to patience and provide the calm, caring environment that both you and your loved one deserve.

Recap: The Virtue of Patience

Patience is like a soft, warm blanket on a chilly night. It's the gentle hand that steadies us when we feel like we can't stand still. In the world of caregiving, especially for those with dementia, patience isn't just a nice thing to have; it's as crucial as the very air we breathe. But why is it so important, you ask? Let's take a moment and think about it together.

When we care for someone with dementia, we step into a world that moves at a much different pace than we're used to. Things that once took moments might now take minutes or hours. It can be hard, really hard. But here's the thing: every single second of patience we offer is a gift of love to the person we're caring for. It tells them, "You are important to me, and I will wait for you." Isn't that beautiful?

So, what have we learned about patience in this journey together, and how can we wrap it up in a way that sticks with you, giving you something solid to hold onto? Here's a step-by-step guide for all of us:

Embrace the Pace: Understand that in dementia care, things slow down. And that's okay. It doesn't mean we're not making progress. • Set Realistic Expectations: Know that victories come in all sizes. Sometimes, a small step is just as valuable as a big leap. • Communicate with Care: Always speak with kindness and give the person with dementia the time they need to respond. • Patience in Routine: Work patience into your daily tasks. Whether it's mealtime or a walk in the park, let the pace be slow if it needs to be. • Keep Your Cool: When you start to feel impatient, take a deep breath. Remember why you're doing this. You are making a difference.

Now, let's dive deeper and really understand each of these steps, shall we? First, embracing the pace means accepting the new tempo of our loved ones' lives. We allow ourselves to slow down, step by step, to match their rhythm. And when we do that, we're not just waiting; we're being present. That's a gift not only to them but to ourselves too.

Next, setting realistic expectations is about being honest with ourselves. Sure, we all wish for quick progress. But in dementia care, the small moments, like a smile or remembering a name, are the big wins. Celebrate them and cherish them.

Clear and patient communication is about more than words. It's about body language, it's about tone of voice, and it's about giving the person the time they need to process and respond. This tells them, "I'm here, and I'm listening.

Patience in daily routines might seem like a small thing, but it's huge. It's the difference between a rushed morning that leaves everyone feeling frazzled and a calm start to the day that sets a peaceful tone for both of you. And when it comes to keeping your cool, remember this: your feelings are valid.

It's natural to feel impatient sometimes. But finding ways to cope with those feelings, like deep breathing or stepping away for a moment, helps us come back to our caregiving role with renewed patience.

We've talked a lot about patience, haven't we? But it's for a good reason: Patience is powerful. It builds trust, it forms bonds, and it brings peace. And in a world that often feels like it's racing by, patience is our way of saying, "I choose to walk this journey at a pace that's right for us, no matter how slow or fast that might be."

So, dear caregiver, as we wrap up this chat, remember the power of patience. Hold onto it, practice it, and let it guide you through the ups and downs of caregiving. It's not just about being patient with the person you're caring for; it's about being patient with yourself too. You're doing an incredible job, and every moment of patience is a step forward, for both of you.

Thank you for taking the time to talk about patience in caregiving. Hold onto these steps, use them, and watch how they can change your caregiving journey for the better. Patience is truly a virtue, and in your hands, it becomes a source of strength and love. Now, let's keep going, step by patient step, together.

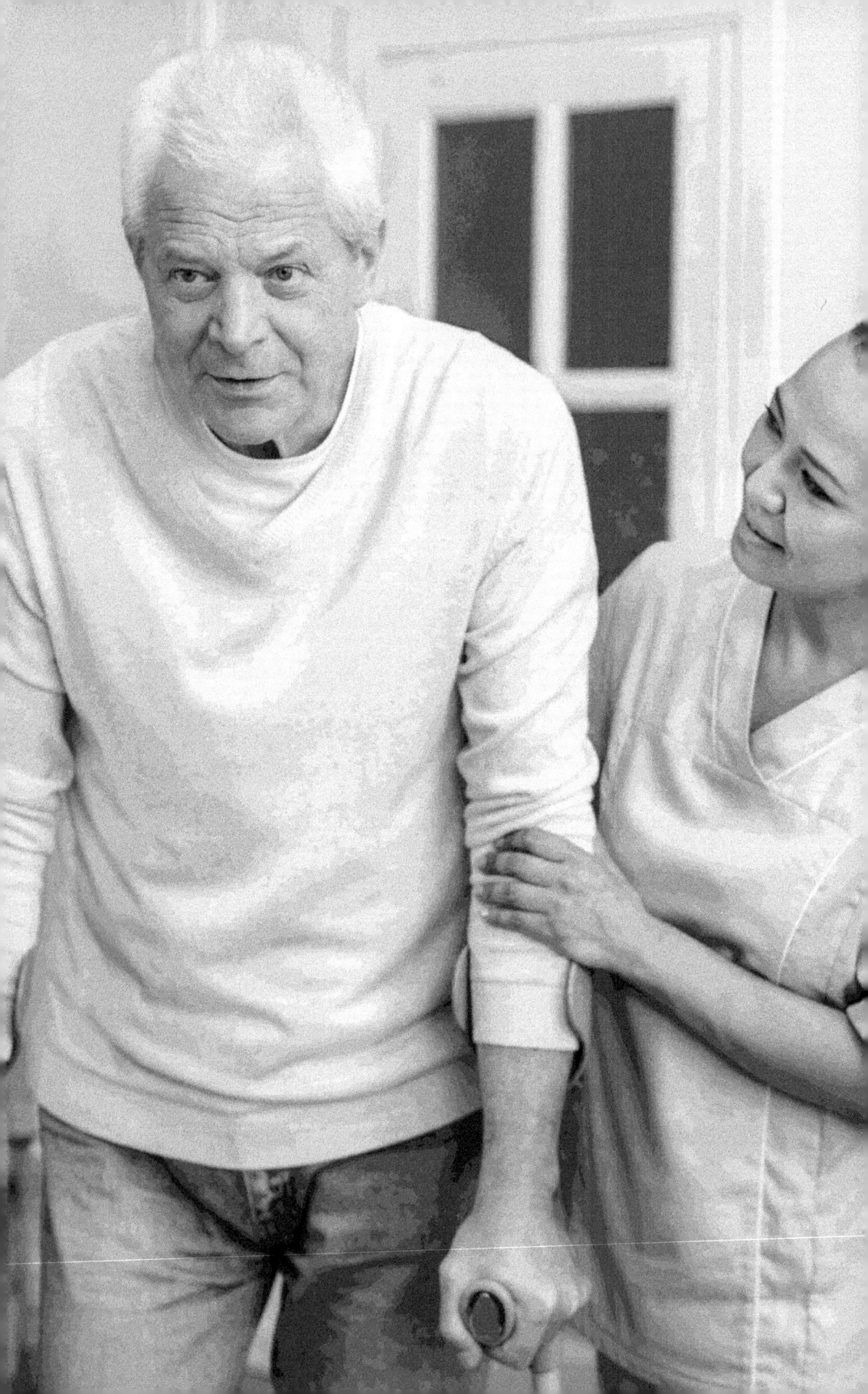

Chapter Five.
Adaptability in Caregiving

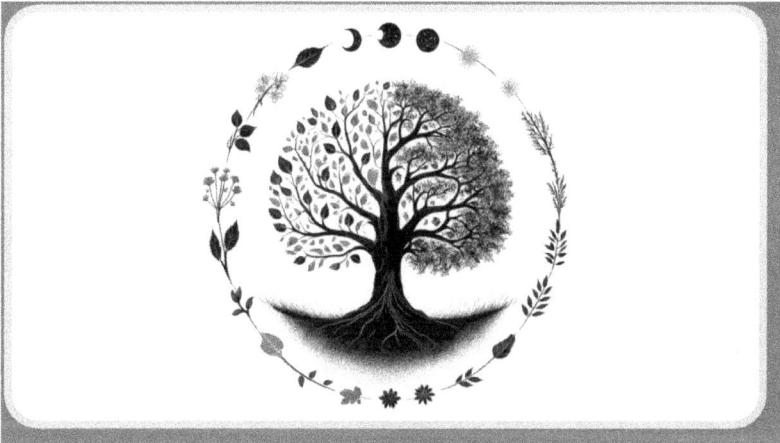

"The longer I live the more beautiful life becomes."

– Frank Lloyd Wright

Navigating the Unpredictable

Adaptiblity. It's a word that sounds simple, but when it comes to dementia care, it's a powerful skill. It's all about being ready for anything that might happen. When you care for someone with dementia, things can change very fast. One day, things might be calm. The next day could be very different. It can be hard, but you can do it. And I am here to help you learn how.

What Does Adaptability in Dementia Care Mean?

It's about staying calm when things change. It's about thinking fast and finding new ways to help your loved one. Your mom or dad, your grandparent, or a friend may not act the same way every day. Their needs could change. They might forget things, or they might get upset for no reason you can see. You need to understand that this can happen. You need to be ready to help in a new way.

Why is this important? When you can change what you do to help, you can make life better for the person you care for. They feel safer and happier. And you can feel good about finding ways to help them, even when it's tough. You become a better caregiver when you can change your plans to fit what's happening right now. This might mean doing things differently from how you did them before. But that's okay. You're learning. And every time you learn something new, you get better at caring for your loved one.

How Do You Stay Ahead of Changes?

One way is to watch and listen. Pay close attention to the person you're helping. Notice little things. Maybe they can't find the right words today. Maybe they don't want to eat what they usually love. These small signs can tell you something is different. When you see these signs, think about what they might need. Maybe they need you to talk slower. Maybe they need a different food. Maybe they just need you to sit with them and hold their hand.

Watching and listening help you understand what's happening. But there's more you can do. You can also learn about dementia. Read books. Talk to doctors. Join groups where people share their stories. The more you know, the better you can be ready for what might come. You learn from what other people have seen and done. You learn about the ways dementia can change how people act and feel. This knowledge is like a tool. You can use it to help you decide what to do when things change.

Being ready for change also means taking care of yourself. When you feel good and have energy, it's easier to handle surprises. Make sure to get some rest. Eat healthy food. Find time to relax. Talk to friends. Laugh. When you care for yourself, you have more to give to the person with dementia. You can think more clearly. You're more patient. You can smile even when things are hard. This makes a big difference for you and the person you're helping.

When things change, you might feel scared or unsure. That's normal. But remember, you're not alone. Many people have walked this path before you. They've learned how to adapt. They've found ways to make each day a good one, no matter what happens. And you can learn this too. Every day you care for someone with dementia, you're getting stronger. You're learning more. You're becoming a hero on this journey. And that's something very special.

Now, let's think about what you can do today. Look at the person you're helping. See how they're doing. Are they happy? Are they confused? What do they need? Then think about what you can do to help them feel better. Maybe you can play their favorite song. Maybe you can show them pictures and talk about old times. Maybe you just need to sit quietly with them. Try different things. See what works. And don't worry if you need to try again. That's how you learn.

Every time you try something new and it works, you're winning. You're making life better for someone you care about. And that's a beautiful thing. You might not get it right every time, but that's okay. The fact that you're trying is what matters. You're showing love and care. And that's the most important part of being a caregiver.

Anticipating Change

Caregiving, at its heart, is about helping someone you care about. Sometimes, the person you're caring for might have dementia. Dementia can make things tough. It changes how a person thinks and acts. This means that if you're taking care of someone with dementia, you need to be ready for things to change a lot.

Now, you might be thinking, "How can I get ready for something if I don't know what's going to happen?" That's a good question. Let me tell you, being ready is all about thinking ahead. It's like when you pack an umbrella because it might rain. You don't know if it will rain for sure, but you're ready just in case.

So, here's what you can do to get ready for the changes that might come with dementia care. The first thing is to watch and learn. Pay close attention to the person you're helping. Notice the small things. How did they act yesterday? What did they eat? Did they sleep well? By paying attention, you'll start to see patterns. You might see that they get upset before dinner. Or they might have trouble sleeping after watching TV.

Once you see these patterns, you can make small changes that help a lot. Maybe you give them a snack before dinner so they're not too hungry. Or you might read a book with them instead of watching TV before bed. These small steps can make a big difference.

Another way to be ready is to talk to people who know about dementia. This could be a doctor, a nurse, or other caregivers. They can tell you about the kinds of changes to expect. They can also give you tips on how to handle different situations. It's like having a map when you're going on a trip. It shows you the way and helps you get ready for the journey.

There's another important part of getting ready for change, and that's taking care of yourself. When you're strong and healthy, you can handle change better. This means eating right, getting enough sleep, and taking breaks when you need them. Think of it like putting on your own oxygen mask before helping others on an airplane. You have to be okay to help someone else be okay.

And remember, it's okay to ask for help. Caregiving is a big job, and it's fine to reach out to friends, family, or support groups. They can give you a break, help you out, or just listen when you need to talk. It's like having a team in a sport. You work together to win the game.

So, to sum up, getting ready for change when you're taking care of someone with dementia means paying attention, learning from others, taking care of yourself, and asking for help when you need it. By doing these things, you'll be able to adjust your care as things change. And that's a big part of being a good caregiver.

When you're ready for what might come, you can keep calm and help the person you care for feel safe and loved. That's what really matters. And when you can do that, you're doing an amazing job as a caregiver, no matter what changes come your way.

Strategies for Adaptation

When caring for someone with dementia, every day can bring new surprises. The way things were yesterday might not be the way they are today. And that's okay. We are here to learn how to turn every twist into a chance to get better at what we do. To give the best care possible, we need to be ready to change our plans and learn from what happens.

First off, let's talk about what it means to adapt. When we adapt, we change to fit new conditions. Think about a tree. When the wind blows, the tree bends. It doesn't break; it moves with the wind and then stands tall again when it's calm. We need to be like the tree. Bend, but don't break. Move with the changes, not against them.

So, how can we do this? It starts with an open mind. When we wake up each day, let's tell ourselves, "Today may be different, and that's going to be okay." We need to be willing to change our routines if we need to. If our loved one is having a tough day, we might need to slow down and take it easy. Or maybe they are full of energy, and we need to find more activities to keep them busy.

One way to adapt is to make a care plan, but not just any plan. Our plan needs to have room for change. Think about having a few different activities ready to go. If one thing doesn't work out, we can try another. It's like having a box of tools. We can pick the right tool for the job depending on the problem we need to solve.

Something else we can do is watch and learn. We can watch how our loved ones act and what they like or don't like. Maybe they smile when they hear music. We can remember that and play music when they seem down. Paying attention to these little things can help us a lot. We learn what works and what doesn't, and we use that knowledge to do better every day.

Let's not forget to talk to others, too. There are people out there who have been taking care of their loved ones for a long time. They have seen a lot and learned a lot. We can ask them for advice. What do they do when things get hard? What has helped them the most? Their stories can teach us new ways to handle our own challenges.

Another important strategy is to take breaks. When we're tired, it's hard to think straight. We need to rest so we can be our best for our loved ones. Taking a short walk or sitting quietly for a few minutes can help us clear our minds. Then we can come back and see things in a new way. A fresh mind can spot new solutions to problems.

Lastly, we have to be kind to ourselves. Sometimes, things will not go as planned. We might feel like we've failed. But that's not true. We are doing our best, and that's all anyone can do. When things get tough, we need to remind ourselves that we are learning and growing. Every day is a new chance to get better.

In the end, adapting is all about learning. We try something, and if it doesn't work, we try something else. We keep doing this, and over time, we get really good at caring for our loved ones. We become like the tree that bends with the wind. Strong, flexible, and always ready for what comes next.

Now, you've got some strategies to help you adapt. Remember, every challenge is a chance to learn. Watch, listen, ask, rest, and be kind to yourself. Use these tools, and you'll be able to handle anything that comes your way.

Learning from Each Experience

When we think about caring for someone, each day can be like a new page in a big book. It's full of surprises. Some days are good and some days are not so good. But every day, there's something new to learn. That's what this part is all about. Learn from every day with your loved one who has dementia. Let's dive into why this is so important.

See, when we learn from what happens each day, we get better at caring. We start to understand little things. When is the best time to eat? Or what makes your loved one happy? Or when they need quiet time? Every little thing you notice is like a gold coin you put in your pocket. It helps you be ready for what comes next.

Sometimes you might feel like you're not doing well. Maybe something you tried didn't work. It's okay. We all have those moments. The key is to think about what happened. Ask yourself, "What can I learn from this?" It could be something small. Like learning that loud noises make your loved one upset. So next time, you can make things quieter. Every experience, even the hard ones, teaches us something.

Why is this learning so important, you ask? Well, it helps us adapt. When you know more, you can do better. You can find new ways to help your loved one feel safe and happy. And when they feel better, you feel better too. It's like when you learn to ride a bike. At first, you might fall. But then you learn how to balance. And soon, you're riding without even thinking about it. That's how it is with caregiving too.

Let's talk about some steps to help you learn from each experience: First, take note of things each day. You could write them down or just remember them. Little things like "Dad smiled when we listened to his favorite song" or "Mom was calm when we looked at old pictures." These notes are like a map. They show you what works.

Next, try new things. If you see that something is not making your loved one happy, change it. Try a different activity or a new way to talk to them. It's like when you're cooking. If you add too much salt once, next time, you add less. You cook, you taste, and you learn.

Another step is to share with others. Talk to friends or people who also care for someone. They might have good tips for you. It's like sharing recipes. Someone else's idea could be just what you need. And your ideas could help someone else too!

Then, make a little time for yourself. Think about your day. Were there hard moments? Were there good moments? What made them that way? When you think about these things, it's like putting puzzle pieces together. You start to see the whole picture of what caring for your loved one is like.

Last, don't be hard on yourself. Learning takes time. Remember, every day is a new chance to learn something new. It's a journey. And like any journey, there will be bumps in the road. But each bump teaches you something. And before you know it, you're cruising down the road, feeling more sure about what you're doing.

So, keep your eyes open and your mind ready to learn. Every single day with your loved one is a chance to learn. It's a gift. And when you learn, you become a better caregiver. Your loved one feels it. And they feel better too. It's a beautiful thing, this learning. It makes the hard work of caregiving a little bit easier. And a lot more rewarding.

In the end, we all want to do our best for our loved ones and for ourselves. Learning from each experience is how we get there. It's how we grow. It's how we turn every challenge into a chance to be better. And that's something truly amazing.

So let's keep learning. Let's keep caring. And let's make each day a little better than the one before. Together, we can do this. And remember, you're not alone. Others are on this journey too. And we're all learning together. That's the beauty of caregiving. It connects us. It teaches us. And it helps us give the best care we can.

Embracing Flexibility

Caregiving is a journey. It's a path that twists and turns, with every day bringing something new. A caregiver needs to be ready for anything. Let's talk about adaptability. It's like having a backpack full of tools. You might not know which tool you'll need, but you're prepared to dig in and find the right one when the time comes. Flexibility is one of those essential tools in your caregiving backpack. It's not just about being able to touch your toes! It's about the heart and the mind. It's about bending without breaking.

Flexibility in caregiving means having a soft heart and an open mind. It means that when your loved one wakes up and today is not like yesterday, you take a deep breath. You smile. You adjust. You find a new way to make today a good one. It starts with small steps. Building a flexible care strategy isn't a race. It's more like gardening. You plant seeds. You water them. You watch them grow. You deal with weeds and pests. And you adapt to the weather.

First, we look at the plan. A care plan is like a map. It shows you where you are and where you want to go. But sometimes the roads are closed. Sometimes, you need to find a new route. This is okay. This is expected. In caregiving, we learn to redraw our maps. We learn to enjoy the scenery along the detour. The new route might even be better. It might have something beautiful to see that you would have missed otherwise.

When we embrace flexibility, we look out for changes. We expect them. We welcome them. It's like being a weather watcher. You can see the clouds gathering. You feel the air change. You know a storm might be coming. You don't get upset. You don't wish for sun when rain is on the horizon. You just get out the umbrella. Maybe you even splash in the puddles. Changes in your loved one's behavior or needs are those clouds. You can be ready with an umbrella.

Being flexible means learning as you go. It's not about being perfect. It's about trying and seeing what works and what doesn't. It's like playing a game where the rules change. You might not win every round. That's not the point. The point is to keep playing, to keep enjoying the game. Every day with your loved one is a chance to learn new rules, play a new round, and find joy in playing.

Now, let's talk about those steps to implementing a flexible care strategy. It's not hard. It's like learning to dance. At first, you might step on a few toes. But soon, you will find the rhythm. You find your feet moving in time to the music. You start to feel the joy of the dance.

Step one is to listen. Listen to your loved one. They might not use words. They might use sounds. They might use movements. But they're speaking. Listen with your ears, your eyes, and your heart. What are they telling you? What do they need today? Tomorrow? Listening is the first step in dancing. It's how you find the beat.

Step two is to learn. Every day is a lesson. What worked? What didn't? Keep a journal. Write it down. This is your dance card. It shows you which steps were graceful, and which were clumsy. It helps you plan for the next dance. Learning in caregiving is like adding new steps to your routine. Every day, you're a better dancer than you were the day before.

Step three is to let go. Let go of what you thought the day would be. Let go of the perfect routine. Embrace the unexpected. It's like improv theater. You're given a prompt, and you make up the scene as you go. The audience is your loved one. They don't care if you miss a line. They're just happy to be part of the show. Letting go is freeing. It allows you to move with the moment, to create something unique and special.

Step four is to love. Love the process. Love the moments, even the hard ones. Love your loved ones, just as they are. Caregiving is an act of love. It's a daily affirmation of that love. Flexibility is the expression of that love. It says, "I am here for you, however you are today, whatever you need today." Loving in caregiving is like singing a lullaby. It's soothing, it's comforting, and it's filled with love.

Finally, step five is to live. Live in the moment. Live for joy. Live for the love. Caregiving is not just about giving care. It's about sharing a life. It's about making memories, even in the midst of challenges. Living in caregiving is like throwing a party. It doesn't matter if the cake is lopsided or if the decorations are falling down. What matters is the laughter, the stories, and the connection.

So there you have it. Steps to embrace flexibility. Listen, learn, let go, love, and live. It's a dance. It's a song. It's a play. It's a party. It's caregiving. When you embrace flexibility, you're not just a caregiver. You're a listener, a learner, a player, a lover, and a liver of life. Isn't that a wonderful thing to be?

When you walk away from this, remember the steps. They're simple, but they're profound. They'll help you be the caregiver you want to be. They'll help you give the care your loved one deserves. Listen, learn, let go, love, and live. With these steps, you're ready. Ready to dance in the rain, ready to learn new steps, ready to love with all your heart, and ready to live a life filled with caregiving joy. You're ready for the journey. Now, take that first step.

Recap: The Adaptive Caregiver

We've talked a lot about the ups and downs in the life of a caregiver. Now, it's time to wrap up what we've learned about being change-ready. Being a caregiver for someone with dementia is like sailing a boat on ever-changing seas. You need to be ready to move with the waves, steer through storms, and enjoy the calm when it comes. That's what being adaptable is all about. It's not just a nice skill to have; it's essential.

So, why is adaptability so important? Here's the thing. When you care for someone with dementia, things change a lot. What works today might not work tomorrow. The person you care for may feel one way now and very different soon after. Your role is to be there, steady, and ready to change your approach whenever needed. This can mean switching up daily routines, changing how you communicate, or finding new activities that bring joy. It's all part of the journey.

Now, how do you develop this super skill of adaptability? It's a mix of mindset and action. Let's look at some steps you can take to become an adaptable caregiver:

- **Stay Informed**: Keep learning about dementia. Knowledge is power, and the more you know, the better you can adapt.

- **Plan Ahead**: Have a plan, but know it's just a starting point. Always be ready to change that plan.

- **Reflect**: After each day, think about what worked and what didn't. Use this info to do better next time.

- **Be Open**: Listen to the person you're caring for. Really listen. They'll show you how you need to adapt.

- **Take Care of Yourself**: You can't be adaptable if you're worn out. Rest, recharge, and then you can give your best.

- **Get Support**: Talk to other caregivers. Share

stories and advice. You're not alone on this journey.

- **Stay Positive**: A sunny outlook can make adaptability much easier. Believe that you can handle the changes.

- **Practice**: Adaptability is like a muscle. The more you use it, the stronger it gets. Keep practicing.

Now let's dive deeper into each of these steps. When you stay informed, you're arming yourself with the best tool: knowledge. Read books, attend workshops, and talk with professionals. Learn about the stages of dementia and what might come your way. It's like having a map for your journey. You might take some unexpected paths, but you'll know the terrain.

Planning is not about setting a strict schedule. It's more like sketching a rough outline. You know things will change, but having a plan gives you a place to start. When change happens, take a deep breath. Look at your plan.

What can you adjust? Maybe it's time for a meal or activity to change. That's okay. The plan was just your first draft.

Reflecting on your day is like being your own coach. Ask yourself, What worked? What didn't? Why? Maybe you tried a new activity that made the person you care for smile. Great! Let's do that again. Maybe something upsets them. Alright, let's avoid that next time. Take notes if it helps. It's all important information for your adaptability toolkit.

Being open means truly hearing what the person with dementia is saying, with words and actions. Maybe they're more talkative in the morning. Maybe they get upset with too much noise. Listen, learn, and adapt. Their needs are your guide.

Taking care of yourself is not selfish. It's necessary. If you're tired or stressed, you won't be able to adapt as well. Get enough sleep, eat well, and find time for yourself. Even a short break can make a big difference. When you're at your best, you can give your best care.

Getting support is like finding teammates. Other caregivers can share their own adaptability tips and tricks. Join a support group or find an online community. Swap stories and learn from each other. It's comforting to know others are riding the same waves.

A positive attitude will be your anchor. Believe in yourself and your ability to handle changes. Every day might bring something new, but you've got this. Your positive energy can even rub off on the person you're caring for. Smiles are contagious, after all.

Lastly, practice makes perfect. Well, maybe not perfect, but it makes you better. Every time you adapt, you get a little bit better at it. Like learning to dance, at first, you might step on a few toes, but soon you'll be gliding across the floor.

So there you have it. Being an adaptive caregiver is about staying on your toes and being ready to shift and sway as needed. It's about learning from each day and each moment. In the world of caregiving, change is the only constant. Embrace it, and you'll do more than just manage; you'll thrive. And isn't that what we all want?

To not only get through the day but to make each day as good as it can be, for ourselves and for those we care for. Being adaptable doesn't mean you have to do it all alone, either. Reach out, connect, and keep growing. And when you look back, you'll see how far you've come. You'll see a path marked with challenges, yes, but also victories, big and small. Each one is a step forward. Each one is a reason to keep going. And that, my friend, is what being an adaptive caregiver is all about.

Chapter Six.
Tenderness in Dementia Care

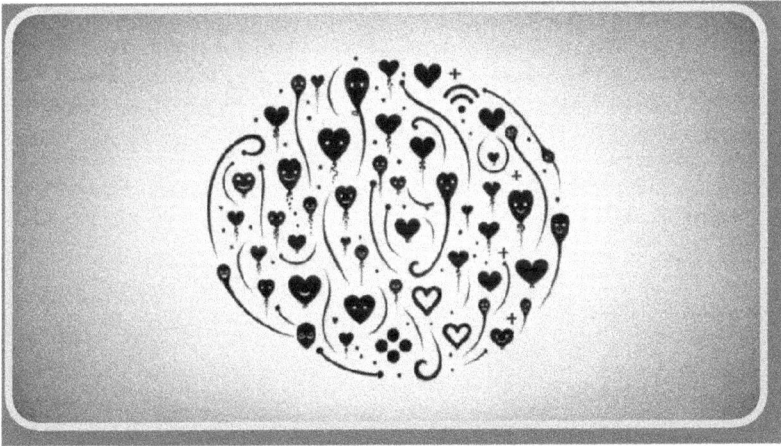

"Too often we underestimate the power of a touch, a smile, a kind word, a listening ear, an honest compliment, or the smallest act of caring, all of which have the potential to turn a life around."

– Leo Buscagli

The Healing Power of Tenderness

When we think of tenderness; we often picture a soft touch or a gentle word. But in the world of caregiving, especially for those with dementia, tenderness is much more. It's a powerful tool that can heal both the body and the mind.

Tenderness in caregiving is about more than just being nice. It's about making a real connection with someone. It means showing them love and care in a way that they can feel, even if they can't say it back to you. And it's not just a feeling; it's backed by science and psychology. Scientists have looked into this, and they tell us that when we give care with tenderness, it can lead to some pretty amazing things. For example, when a caregiver is tender, the person with dementia might feel calmer and happier. They might even sleep better and get along more with others. And it's not just good for the person with dementia; the caregiver feels better, too. They might not feel as stressed or tired.

Now, let's talk about why this happens. When someone is tender with us, it makes our brain release certain chemicals. These chemicals, like oxytocin, are like little messengers that tell our bodies to relax and feel safe. It's like getting a warm hug from the inside. For someone with dementia, these feelings are very important. They can help them feel less scared and confused.

Let's think about what this looks like in real life. Picture helping someone with their meal. If we do this with tenderness, we might take the time to sit with them, talk to them, and make sure they're comfortable. We're not just feeding them; we're sharing a moment with them. And this can make a big difference in how they feel about mealtime and about us.

In daily caregiving situations, tenderness can turn a routine task into an opportunity for connection. Bathing someone might not seem like a special time, but if we do it with tenderness, it can be calming and reassuring for the person. We make sure the water is just right, we speak softly, and we ensure they feel respected and cared for.

What's really interesting is that tenderness doesn't just help in the moment. It can also have long-term effects. When we're consistently tender in our care, the person with dementia may start to trust us more. They feel loved and valued. This can make a big difference in their overall well-being.

But it's not just about the person receiving care. Being tender can also change the caregiver. It can remind us why we do this important work. It can make us feel proud and happy to help someone else. And that feeling can keep us going on tough days.

So, what can we take away from all this? Being tender isn't just a nice thing to do; it's a powerful way to care for someone with dementia. It helps them feel better, and it helps us feel better, too. And that's a win-win for everyone.

When we finish our day of caregiving, we can look back and know that we did more than just our job. We made someone's life a little brighter and a little better. And that's something truly special. And remember, this isn't just talk. This is real. This is something you can do. Every day, with every small act of care, you can bring the healing power of tenderness to someone who needs it. And that's a pretty amazing thing to be able to do.

So, keep this in mind as you care for others. Let tenderness be your guide. And watch as it transforms the caregiving experience for both you and the person you're helping. It's not always easy, but it's always worth it. And that's the truth.

Expressing Tenderness

When caring for someone with dementia, showing tenderness is more than just a kind act. It's a powerful way to connect. Tenderness can be shown in many ways. It's in the gentle way you touch their hand. It's in the warm tone of your voice when you speak. And it's in the little actions you take every day to make their lives better.

Touch is a basic human need. It can speak louder than words. For someone with dementia, a kind touch can be very calming. It can be as simple as a pat on the back or holding their hand. This kind of touch is important. It makes people feel safe and loved.

The way you talk to someone also matters a lot. A soft and friendly voice can soothe and comfort. When you talk to someone with dementia, use a tone that shows you care. This helps them feel understood and respected. It's not just about the words you choose, but how you say them.

Tenderness is also in your actions. It's doing things with a kind heart. This can mean taking the time to listen. Or it can mean being patient when they are confused. It could be making their favorite meal. Or setting up a space where they can enjoy their hobbies. It's all about making their day a little brighter.

Every day, you have chances to be tender. It could be when you help them get dressed. Or when you're making meals. It could be during bath time or when you're helping them move around. These are all times when you can show them they matter.

Your approach to showing tenderness should fit the person you are caring for. Everyone is different. Some people like hugs. Others might not like to be touched too much. You need to learn what makes them feel good. And then do those things. This shows you respect their needs and likes.

All of this takes time and thought. But it's worth it. When you show tenderness, you make life better for the person with dementia. You help them feel understood and cared for. And that is a very special thing to do.

To show tenderness well, you also need to know yourself. You must be aware of your own feelings. Sometimes you might feel tired or upset. That's okay. It's normal. But it's important to take care of yourself too. When you are okay, you can give better care to others.

It's not always easy to be tender. But it's a choice you can make. Choose to show love and care every day. And remember, the little things you do can mean a lot. They can make a big difference in someone's life. And that can make you feel good too.

So, take a moment each day to think. Think about how you can show tenderness. It could be a kind word. A gentle touch. A patient's ear. Find ways to show you care. And do them with all your heart. Don't forget, that being tender is not just good for the person with dementia. It's good for you, too. It can make you feel happy and proud. Proud of the care you give and happy to make a difference in someone's life.

Now, here's something you can do. Try to smile more. Smiling is a simple way to show tenderness. It can make someone's day better. And it doesn't cost anything. Showing tenderness is a beautiful part of caregiving. It's something that can make a big change. It can turn a regular day into a special one. And it can change a hard moment into a warm memory. So, let's choose to be tender. Let's show that we care. Every single day.

Tenderness and Communication

Caregiving is a journey, a path where every step matters and every gesture counts. Imagine a bridge that connects two worlds: the one of the caregiver and the one of the person with dementia. This bridge is built from the bricks of communication, held together by the mortar of tenderness. It's not just words that we exchange; it's a profound connection that we establish.

It's simple, really. When you talk to someone with tenderness, you don't just speak; you reach out with your heart. You let the person know that they are not alone and that you are there with them every step of the way. It's in the tone of your voice, the look in your eyes. It's in the patience you show when words escape them and the gentle way you guide the conversation back on track.

Now, communication is not just about talking. It's about listening, too. When someone has dementia, their words might get jumbled, but the feelings behind those words are clear. Listen. Really listen. Not just for words, but for emotions, for the unspoken needs that linger in silence. Sometimes, the most tender thing you can do is to be present, to bear witness to their struggle, and to acknowledge their efforts to connect.

So, how do we enhance our verbal and non-verbal communication with empathy? Let's focus on verbal first. It starts with slowing down. Speak in a calm, soft voice. Choose your words with care. Use simple sentences. This is not about dumbing things down; it's about clarity. It's respecting the processing time of the person with dementia, giving them the space to understand and respond.

Non-verbal communication is equally, if not more, powerful. It's the warmth of a smile, the comfort of a gentle touch. A nod to encourage them to keep speaking. It's creating a safe space with your body language. Stand or sit at their level: Make eye contact if they are comfortable with it. Be there, fully, with your whole being. It shows, and it matters.

Overcoming personal barriers to expressing tenderness isn't always easy. You might be having a hard day, or you might not naturally show your emotions. But remember, showing tenderness is a choice, a conscious decision to put the needs of the person with dementia first. It's finding that softness in your heart, that patience, and that kindness, and letting it shine through in your actions and words.

Often, we think we need to fill the silence, but sometimes the most tender thing we can do is to allow for quiet. To sit together, to hold a hand, to simply be. It's okay if you don't have the right words. Your presence is a powerful message of love and support, and sometimes it speaks louder than words ever could.

Keep in mind, that every day is different. Some days, communication flows like a gentle stream. Other days, it's a puzzle, a maze of confusion. But with a heart full of tenderness, you adapt. You adjust your approach. You learn the dance of back and forth, of give and take, of speaking and listening. And through it all, you never lose sight of the person behind the disease.

Finally, remember to take care of yourself, too. You can't pour from an empty cup. Find ways to recharge, to fill your own well of tenderness, so that you can continue to share it with others. Whether it's a walk in the park, a cup of tea in the quiet of the early morning, or a chat with a friend, find what nourishes your soul. It's essential. Because when you take care of yourself, you can take better care of others.

So, take a moment to reflect. How can you incorporate more tenderness into your communication today? Start small. A kind word, a listening ear, a moment of patience. It adds up; it makes a difference. And remember, this isn't just about the person with dementia. It's about you, too. It's about building a world where tenderness is the language we all speak fluently and where every interaction is an opportunity for connection, compassion, and care.

Let's create a ripple effect of tenderness, starting with our words and actions, reaching the heart of the person with dementia, and extending out into the world.

It's a beautiful journey, and it starts with you. Keep going, keep caring, and keep communicating with tenderness. It's the most precious gift you can give, and the rewards are immeasurable.

Overcoming Barriers to Tenderness

When you care for someone with dementia, being tender is like giving them a warm blanket in the cold. It feels good, right? But some days, it's hard to be tender. You may feel tired or upset. It's not just you. Many people feel this way. Caregivers often have a lot of stress. They get worn out. It's normal. So, what can you do?

First, let's talk about stress. Stress is like a heavy backpack. When you're stressed, it's like carrying a backpack filled with rocks. It makes everything harder. Stress can make it tough to be gentle and tender. But it's important to try. Why? Because tenderness can help the person you're caring for feel safe and loved. And that's a big deal.

Now, let's think about what makes you stressed. Is it too much work? Not enough sleep? Or maybe you feel sad about the person's dementia. It's okay to have these feelings. The key is to know what they are. Once you know, you can start to make things better. How? By taking care of yourself.

Self-care is like putting on your oxygen mask first on a plane. You have to help yourself before you can help others. So, take breaks when you need them. Eat good food. Try to sleep well. Maybe talk to a friend or go for a walk. These things can help you feel better. When you feel better, it's easier to be tender and kind.

Another thing that can get in the way is emotional fatigue. Emotional fatigue is feeling too tired inside to care. It happens when you give a lot of yourself for a long time. When you're emotionally tired, being tender can feel impossible. What can you do? First, know that it's okay to feel this way. You're not alone. Many caregivers feel the same. Second, ask for help. Maybe a friend or family member can take over for a bit. Just a little time off can help you recharge.

It's also good to have a way to let out your feelings. Maybe you can write in a journal or talk to someone who understands. When you let your feelings out, they don't weigh you down as much. And that can make it easier to show tenderness again.

Now let's talk about something really important: self-awareness. Self-awareness is like knowing the map of your heart. It means understanding your feelings. When you're self-aware, you can see when stress or sadness is coming, and you can do something before it gets too big.

How do you become more self-aware? You can start by stopping a few times a day to ask yourself, "How am I feeling right now?" Just this simple question can help you see what's going on inside. And when you know what's going on, you can take steps to feel better. Like taking a break or doing something fun.

Another helpful thing is self-regulation. This is like driving a car with good brakes. It means being able to slow down or stop when your feelings get too strong. Say you're feeling really upset. Self-regulation is taking a deep breath and counting to ten. It's a way to calm down before you say or do something you might regret. Also, it helps you stay tender and gentle, even when it's hard.

What about those really tough days? The days when nothing seems to go right? It's hard, but you can still be tender. One way to do this is to think about why you're a caregiver. Maybe you're doing it because you care about the person. Remembering this can give you strength. It can help you be kind, even when it's tough.

And here's a tip: Try to be tender to yourself, too. When we're kind to ourselves, it's easier to be kind to others. So give yourself a break. Tell yourself you're doing a good job. Because you are. Caregiving is hard work. And you're doing it. That's something to be proud of.

Last, let's talk about resilience. Resilience is like being a tree that bends in the wind instead of breaking. It means being able to handle tough times and bounce back. Being resilient can help you keep being tender, even when it's hard. How do you build resilience? By taking care of yourself, asking for help when you need it, and remembering why you're doing this important work.

So, to sum up, being tender is really important in caregiving. But it's not always easy. You can face challenges like stress and emotional fatigue. It's okay to feel this way. The key is to take care of yourself, be aware of your feelings, and ask for help when needed. This can help you keep your heart open and tender. And that's a beautiful gift for the person you're caring for— and for you, too.

Tenderness as a Care Philosophy

Caring for someone with dementia is a journey. It's a path shared by the caregiver and the person with dementia. On this path, the air is often thick with emotions, challenges, and moments of pure connection. To wade through this, we introduce a philosophy. Not just any philosophy, but one rooted in the soft, gentle practice of tenderness.

Tenderness is more than a simple, kind gesture or a warm smile. It is a fundamental approach to caregiving that can transform both the giver and the receiver. Yes, tenderness can change lives. It infuses the care you provide with a kind of warmth that can't be measured by any tool. But let's slow down and talk about this. Let's unpack what it means to make tenderness a cornerstone of your caregiving philosophy.

Let's start with the basics. A philosophy is a way of thinking about something. It's like a pair of glasses that you put on, and they change the way you see things. When you put on the glasses of tenderness, you begin to see the person with dementia not just as a patient but as a person full of stories, emotions, and needs.

But why is this important? Well, imagine a world where every action you take and every word you speak comes from a place of deep kindness. That's the world you create when tenderness guides your care. Over time, this world becomes a safe haven for people with dementia. They feel understood. They feel respected. They feel loved.

Now let's dig deeper. Tenderness doesn't just happen. It's like a garden. You need to plant it, water it, and tend to it. It needs to become a part of who you are when you care for someone. This means always being patient and always being kind, even when the day is long and your spirit is tired. It means speaking with softness and listening with your whole heart, even when words seem to fail. And the benefits? They are as vast as the ocean. When you treat someone with tenderness, their anxiety often melts away. They may become calmer, more cooperative, and even more joyful. But it doesn't stop there. As a caregiver, adopting tenderness as your philosophy can bring you peace. It helps you to forgive yourself on tough days. It reminds you of why you started this journey in the first place.

But how do you build a care environment that reflects tenderness and empathy? It starts with little things. A gentle touch, a warm blanket, or a favorite song can make a world of difference. Creating a routine that allows for slow, tender moments can help the person with dementia feel secure and valued.

Now, let's talk about the long-term benefits. The journey of dementia care is often marked by changes and unknowns. When tenderness is your guide, you create a cushion for these changes. You build a relationship based on trust and affection that can withstand the test of time. For the caregiver, this philosophy can be a source of strength. It can help you connect with your inner wisdom and compassion, making you a better caregiver and a more fulfilled person.

It is essential to remember that tenderness is not a sign of weakness. It is a sign of strength. It takes courage to be gentle in a world that sometimes seems to value toughness. But in the world of dementia care, tenderness is a mighty force. It breaks down walls. It builds bridges. It turns moments of care into moments of love.

So, how do you start integrating tenderness into your caregiving philosophy? First, pay attention to your actions and words. Are they soft? Are they kind? Next, listen to the person with dementia. Really listen. Let them tell you what they need, even if it's not with words. Then, reflect on your day. Did you make space for tenderness? If not, how can you do better tomorrow?

Lastly, remember that tenderness is contagious. When you treat someone with tenderness, it often spreads to others. It can change the whole atmosphere of a place. It can inspire others to be gentle too. And when tenderness spreads, miracles happen. People heal in ways we can't always see. Connections are made that can last a lifetime. It's a beautiful thing.

In conclusion, making tenderness a key element of your care philosophy is not just about doing good. It's about being good. It's about creating a ripple effect of kindness that can transform the world of dementia care. It's about finding joy in the little moments, the quiet moments, and the tender moments. It's about being a light in the life of someone who may sometimes feel lost in the dark. So, take this wisdom with you. Tend to it. Let it grow. And watch as the power of tenderness changes your life and the lives of those you care for. You have the tools now. It's time to use them, to cultivate a caregiving practice that doesn't just exist but thrives with the warmth of tenderness at its heart.

Recap: Cultivating Compassion

We have shared a journey through the depths of tenderness in the care of those with dementia. It's important to pull together the threads of understanding we have gathered. Let's reflect on the significant role tenderness plays in dementia care. This is a journey of the heart, where every small act of kindness echoes in the life of the person you care for.

Tenderness isn't just a feeling; it's a practice, a deliberate choice in how we interact. Whether through a gentle touch or a warm smile, we convey compassion. And it makes a difference. It's about seeing the person, not the disease. It's about connecting with them, where words often fail. This connection is potent. It can turn a routine day into a collection of moments filled with warmth and understanding.

Let us walk through a step-by-step guide, to ensuring tenderness is woven into the daily tapestry of care. These are practical steps that can transform your caregiving routine into an act of love and respect for the person in your care:

1. **Begin each day with a calm heart.** Take deep breaths before you open the door to the room of the person you're caring for. Your peace is the first gift of tenderness you can give.

2. **Meet their eyes with a smile.** No matter how their night was, your smile tells them they're not alone. It's a simple yet profound way to start the day.

3. **Speak softly and kindly.** Use words that soothe, not overwhelm. This is how you set a tone of care and safety that lasts all day.

4. **Listen. Really listen.** When they speak, give them your full attention. Show them that their thoughts and feelings matter to you.

5. **Touch with purpose and gentleness.**

Whether you're helping them dress or simply holding their hand, let your touch be a comfort.

6. **Be patient.** Dementia can make simple tasks challenging. Your patience is a silent message of support and respect for their struggles.

7. **End each encounter with an affirmation.** A warm "See you soon" or "Take care" can be a soothing balm, leaving them with a sense of being cherished.

These steps are more than actions; they are the embodiment of a philosophy of care that celebrates the human spirit despite the trials of dementia.

Now, let's reflect on the transformational power of tenderness. When you care with tenderness, you're not just helping their body; you're healing their soul. You're telling them they're valued. And in this exchange, something remarkable happens. You, the caregiver, are transformed too. Your heart grows. Your capacity for love expands. And the quality of your care reaches new heights.

Remember, tenderness is a gift that benefits both the giver and the receiver. When we care with tenderness, we're building a world that acknowledges the dignity of every person, regardless of their cognitive state. Cultivating compassion isn't just about better care. It's about a better world. It starts in the quiet corners of everyday life, with every tender word and touch. As caregivers, we have the power to make that world real, one act of kindness at a time.

So, take these lessons to your heart. Use them to color your caregiving with the hues of compassion and empathy. And remember, in the world of dementia care, tenderness is not just a nice-to-have; it is essential, it is transformative, it is everything.

And if you're keen to continue growing on this journey, consider joining our community. By subscribing to our newsletter, you become part of a circle of caregivers who share your values. We offer resources, support, and learning opportunities like our 9-Step Calm Caregiving Course and provide even more ways to deepen your understanding and practice of tender care.

Seeking counsel? Our counseling services are there to support you. We understand the journey you're on because we walk it with you. Our workbooks, nurturing articles with audio, and slide videos are designed to complement the care you provide with knowledge and heart.

By becoming a member, you unlock a bundle of products and services tailored for compassionate caregiving. With our resources at your fingertips, you can turn every caregiving challenge into an opportunity for growth and connection. And that's just the beginning. Together, we can create an environment of tenderness that reaches far beyond the walls of any home or care facility. Join us, and let's cultivate compassion, one act of tenderness at a time.

SCAN THIS AND FIND OUT HOW CAREGIVERS
TODAY CAN HELP YOU

Chapter Seven.
Holistic Care Strategies

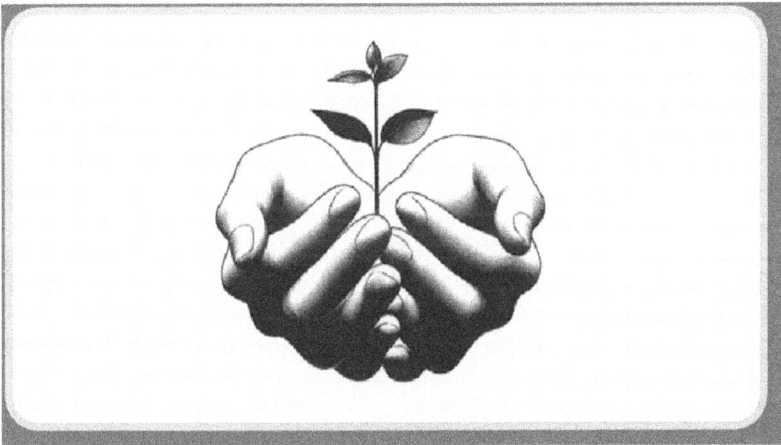

"Nurturing is not complex. It' s merely being tuned in to the thing or person before you and offering small gestures toward what it needs at that time."

– Mary Anne Radmacher

Comprehensive Care for Dementia Patients

When we look after someone with dementia, it's like tending to a garden. Just like flowers need good soil, sunlight, and water, people need care that looks at everything. That's what holistic care is all about. It's caring for the whole garden, not just pulling out the weeds. It's seeing the person, not just the illness. Holistic care wraps around every part of a person's life. This means their body, feelings, and spirit.

Why is this so important? Think about a time when you felt sick. Did you only feel bad in your body? Probably not. Being unwell can make us feel down or worried too. In the same way, when we help someone with dementia, we need to help their whole self.

When we talk about the body, we mean looking after someone's health. We make sure they eat well, move around, and see the doctor. Food is like fuel for our bodies. It keeps us going. Exercise is just as important.

It's like oiling a squeaky door. It helps our bodies work better. And doctors are like gardeners. They keep an eye on our health, making sure we're growing well.

But holistic care doesn't end with the body. Feelings matter too. People with dementia can feel sad, scared, or lonely. We need to listen to them and be there for them. It's like giving water to a thirsty plant. It helps them feel loved and safe.

Then there's the spirit. This isn't just about religion. It's about what makes someone feel alive. It could be music, nature, or being around family. It's like the sunshine in our garden. It helps everything inside us bloom.

So, how do we do this? We start by getting to know the person. What do they like? What matters to them? This helps us make a care plan. It's a map for the garden. It shows us where to plant the flowers and where to build a path. The care plan is our guide. It helps us remember every part of the person's life.

To put the plan together, we talk to the person with dementia, their family, and their doctors. We ask lots of questions. We listen. We write things down. This helps us understand what the person needs.

Now, let's get practical. What can we do today? First, we can make sure the person eats good food. We can cook with them or for them. We can choose foods we like and that are healthy. Next, we can help them move. We can go for walks together or do simple exercises at home. And we can make doctor appointments to check their health.

For their feelings, we can make time to talk. We can share stories and memories. We can hold hands or give hugs. This shows them they're not alone.

For their spirit, we can find activities they enjoy. We can play their favorite music or watch a movie together. We can take them to a park or a church. We find what makes them smile and help them do it more.

Doing all this is a big job. It's like looking after a huge garden. But you don't have to do it alone. You can ask for help. Friends, family, and care professionals can all be part of the team. Each person brings something special. Some might be good at cooking. Others might be great listeners. Together, the team can give the person with dementia the best care.

As a caregiver, it's also important to look after yourself. Remember, you're part of the garden too. If you're not feeling well, it's harder to care for someone else. So take breaks when you need them. Eat well and move your body too. And don't be afraid to ask for help with your feelings or spirit. You're important as well.

Imagine that the garden is now full of color and life. The person with dementia is smiling more. They're eating, moving, and laughing. You're feeling good too.

This is what holistic care can do. It brings out the best in everyone. And it starts with seeing the whole person, not just the illness.

In our next part, we'll dig deeper into each of these areas. We'll learn more about the body, feelings, and spirit. And we'll see how we can grow a garden that's beautiful and healthy, filled with love and care.

Before you go, remember this. Holistic care is a journey, not a race. Take it one step at a time. Keep learning and caring. And watch the garden bloom.

Physical Aspects of Holistic Care

Caring for someone with dementia involves more than remembering to give them their medicine. It is about looking after their whole body. This means thinking about what they eat, how they move, and making sure they see the doctor when they need to. We want to keep them feeling good and strong, not just dealing with their memory problems.

Let's talk about food first. Food is like fuel for our bodies. It gives us the power we need to do everything, from waking up in the morning to going to sleep at night. When someone has dementia, their body needs the right kind of fuel to help them stay as healthy as possible. This means eating lots of foods that are good for them, like fruits, vegetables, whole grains, lean meats, and fish. It's like putting the best gas in a car. The better the fuel, the better the car runs.

But it's not just about what they eat. It's also about enjoying food. We need to make sure the person with dementia likes their food, because if they like it, they will eat more. And when they eat more of the good stuff, their bodies feel better. So we want to find foods that are healthy and yummy.

Exercise is also important. Moving our bodies keeps our muscles and bones strong. It's just like playing. When kids play, they run and jump and feel happy. That's what exercise does for adults, too, even those with dementia. It keeps them moving and happy. We want them to take walks, dance to music, or do simple stretches. Anything that gets them moving in a safe way is great.

Now, we must not forget to take the person with dementia to the doctor for regular check-ups. This is very important. The doctor needs to see them often to make sure everything is working right, just like a mechanic checks a car. The doctor can help fix small problems before they turn into big ones. We want to keep those small problems away, so the person with dementia can have the best days possible.

When we put all these things together—good food, fun exercise, and doctor visits—we help the person with dementia feel good. But it's not just about them feeling good for one day; it's about them feeling good every day. And when they feel good, they can do more things they like. They can smile more, laugh more, and enjoy life more.

We must remember that caring for someone's body is a way of showing love. When we help them eat right, move more, and see the doctor, we are saying, "I care about you." It is a beautiful way to make their life better. And when their lives are better, we feel good too.

So we need to make a plan—a plan that includes healthy foods they like, exercises that are safe and fun, and regular doctor visits. It's like making a list for a big party. We need to think about everything we need to have a great time, and we need to write it down so we don't forget.

But this plan is not just for one day; it's for every day. So we need to keep looking at the plan and making sure we follow it. And sometimes, we need to change the plan. As the person with dementia changes, what they need might change too. So we keep checking and updating the plan to make sure it's always right for them.

In the end, taking care of someone with dementia is about giving them the best life they can have. It's about love and kindness. By taking care of their body with good food, exercise, and doctor's care, we are doing the best we can for them. We are helping them in a big, big way.

Emotional and Spiritual Considerations

Caring for someone with dementia is a journey that stretches beyond just meeting their physical needs. It's about connecting, understanding, and nurturing their emotional and spiritual well-being too. In this section, we will dive deep into how you, as a caregiver, can create a loving environment that speaks to the heart and soul of your loved one.

First, let's talk about emotions. Dementia can be a roller coaster of feelings, not just for those experiencing it but also for those around them. People with dementia often feel lost, confused, and frustrated. They may laugh one minute and cry the next. It's important for caregivers to stay calm and patient. You can help by being a steady presence in their life.

Sometimes, all it takes is a kind word, a gentle touch, or simply being there to listen. Let's focus on listening—really listening. Not just with your ears, but with your heart. Hear not only the words they say but also the emotions they express. When you listen this way, you create a bond—a connection that says, "I'm here for you, and you're not alone."

Let's move on to spiritual support. Spirituality means different things to different people. For some, it's religion. For others, it's a sense of connection to something bigger than themselves. No matter the definition, it's clear that spiritual comfort can be a source of great strength for someone with dementia. So, how do we provide this support? It starts with respect for their beliefs and values. If they find comfort in prayer or religious services, help them continue these practices. It could be as simple as reading holy texts together or playing spiritual music that they love. This can be a soothing and uplifting experience for them.

There's also the power of nature and the great outdoors. Being outside, feeling the sun, and the breeze, and hearing the birds can have a calming effect. It's a way for people with dementia to feel connected to the world around them. Why not take a walk in the park or just sit in the garden? These little moments can mean so much.

Crafting a nurturing environment is about creating a space filled with love and comfort. Fill their room with photos and keepsakes that bring back happy memories. Use soft blankets and pillows to make them feel secure and cozy. Play their favorite music to bring a smile to their face.

Remember, dementia doesn't just affect memory; it touches every part of a person's life. As caregivers, it's our job to make sure we're addressing the whole person, not just the parts that seem the most obvious. It's about making sure they feel seen and valued, not just cared for.

With all of this in mind, I want to leave you with a clear and simple action you can take today. Sit down with your loved one and ask them what brings them joy. What music do they love? What places hold special memories? Use what you learn to create a care plan that includes activities and moments that cater to their emotional and spiritual needs. It's a small step that can make a big difference.

In conclusion, when you take the time to nurture the emotional and spiritual aspects of your loved one's life, you're doing more than just caregiving. You're giving them a sense of belonging, a sense of peace, and a sense of love. And that, my friend, is something truly special.

Social Engagement and Connection

When we consider the care of individuals with dementia, social engagement and connection are often overlooked yet essential pieces of the puzzle. It might seem simple, but it's about more than just keeping someone company. It's about maintaining a person's sense of self, their dignity, and their connections to the world around them.

Humans are social creatures. We need interaction with others to feel alive and like we belong. This doesn't change when someone has dementia. In fact, one could argue that it becomes even more important. Social activities help keep the mind active and engaged. They bring moments of joy and can improve the mood of someone who might feel isolated due to their condition.

So, what are social activities? There are moments when people come together. It could be a family gathering, a group exercise class, or just a simple conversation over a cup of coffee. These activities connect us to the world and to each other, and they can make a huge difference in the life of someone living with dementia.

Now, let's get practical. How do you go about maintaining social interaction for someone with dementia? It's all about understanding the person and finding activities that resonate with their interests and abilities. It could be as simple as looking through family photo albums, listening to their favorite music together, or even watching a beloved TV show. The idea is to create opportunities for engagement that feel natural and enjoyable.

For some, social interaction could be participating in group activities. This could be a painting class, a singing group, or a gentle exercise session tailored to older adults. Group activities are not just fun; they stimulate the mind and can help preserve cognitive functions. They remind the person with dementia that they are part of a community, they are not alone, and they are still valued members of society.

But what if the person with dementia is more introverted? Or what if they find large groups overwhelming? It's important to have one-on-one interactions too.

A caregiver can take on this role by simply having regular conversations. Ask them about their life stories, their hobbies, or their opinions on everyday things. This kind of individual attention can be incredibly comforting and can help maintain a person's language skills.

Now, we know that dementia can make communication challenging. That's why non-verbal activities are just as important. Something as simple as a shared hobby, like gardening, can provide a sense of accomplishment and partnership. Touch, such as holding hands or a gentle hug, can convey love and reassurance when words might fail. Remember, the goal is to maintain a connection, and this can happen in many ways.

What about technology? In our digital age, social engagement can also happen through video calls and social media. This might require a bit of setup and assistance from a caregiver, but imagine the smile on someone's face when they see their grandchild's latest dance recital or hear a distant relative's voice. Technology can bridge gaps and make the world a smaller, friendlier place.

Let's also consider the emotional health benefits of social activities. Being around others can reduce feelings of loneliness and depression, which are common in people with dementia. Laughter, shared stories, and even the occasional shared tears are all parts of a rich tapestry of human experience that shouldn't be denied to anyone, regardless of cognitive ability.

It's also crucial to recognize when social interactions may need to be adjusted. As dementia progresses, the person's ability to engage might change. This requires patience and understanding. The activities that once brought pleasure may no longer have the same effect, and that's okay. It's about adapting and finding new ways to engage and connect.

Lastly, we must not forget that social activities are a two-way street. They also provide respite for caregivers, who can build their support networks and enjoy seeing their loved ones happy. It can be heartwarming to witness moments of clarity and joy, giving a renewed sense of purpose to the caregiving journey.

In conclusion, social engagement and connection play a critical role in caring for someone with dementia. They are about more than just filling time; they are about preserving the essence of a person. By thoughtfully including social activities in a care plan, caregivers can enhance the quality of life for those they care for. And by doing so, they not only support their loved ones but also enrich their own caregiving experience.

Remember, it's the small things that often mean the most. A shared smile, a familiar song, a peaceful moment together. These are the golden threads that weave through the tapestry of care, creating a picture full of warmth, love, and connection. And isn't that what life is all about?

Crafting a Holistic Care Plan

When you create a care plan for someone with dementia, it must be about their whole well-being. This means looking at the person's body, heart, and spirit. We talk about a care plan that fixes all parts of their lives because every part is linked, like pieces of a puzzle that fit together to make the whole picture.

To make a good plan, you first need to know what the person likes and needs. Each person is special. Some love music, while others love walking in the park. The care plan must match what makes them happy and calm. This is important for their happiness and health.

How do we start? We sit down and write all the things that are important for their health. We think about the food they eat, how they move and exercise, and remember to check on their body health with doctor visits. We think about their hearts and the things that make them feel love and joy.

We also remember their spirit—the part of them that needs peace and hope. The next step is to make a list. On the list, we write down every part of their life. We put "food" and list the kinds of food that are good for their brain and body.

We put "move" and write down the activities that keep their bodies strong. We put "doctor" to remember their health checks. We write "love" and list the people and things that make them feel warm inside. We put "hope" and write down the ways they can find peace and comfort.

Now we have a list. But it's not enough to just have a list—we need to turn it into action. We choose things from the list and plan when to do them. Maybe we play their favorite music every morning, plan walks in the park twice a week, and make sure we go to the doctor when it's needed. We plan visits from family or friends that make them smile. We find quiet moments for them to feel peace and think about good things.

As we fill out the plan, we think about balance. We make sure there's time for rest, time for fun, and time for care. We put it all together in a schedule that is not too busy but full of good things.

But we don't do this alone. We talk with the person we are caring for. We ask what they like and want to do—it's their plan, so they should have a say in it. We also talk with other people who care for them. We share ideas and make sure everyone knows the plan and helps to make it work.

When the plan is ready, we start. We do the things we planned and watch carefully to see how the person feels. If they smile more, we'll know it's working. If they seem upset or tired, we change the plan. We learn, and we get better at caring for them.

As time passes, things can change. The person we care for may need different things, so we look at the plan often. We talk about it and update it. This helps the plan stay right for the person as they change.

We also need to take care of ourselves. When we feel good, we can care better for others. So we make sure to rest, eat well, and do things that make us happy too. Taking care of someone is hard work, but when we do it with love and a good plan, it makes a big difference.

Let me tell you, when you see the person you care for laughing or feeling peaceful, it's worth it. It makes all the effort put into making a good plan feel important. And it is important, because in the end, what we all want is to feel good and happy, right?

To wrap it up, creating a care plan is like building a house. We need a strong foundation and good materials, and we need to check on it and fix it when needed. And when we build it with care and love, it becomes a home—a place of comfort and safety.

The same goes for our care plan. We build it with knowledge and love, keep it strong and up-to-date, and make it a source of comfort and safety for the person with dementia. This is how we care for the whole person, not just the disease. It's how we make life better for them and for us.

So, let's do this. Let's make a care plan that brings happiness and health. Let's work together to care for the body, heart, and spirit. And let's remember, in caring for them, we also care for ourselves.

Recap: The Whole Person Approach

Let's step back and look at the journey we've been on together. We've talked a lot about caring for someone with dementia. It's important to remember that care is more than just making sure someone eats and sleeps right. It's about looking at the whole person. This means their body, their feelings, and their spirit too. It's like when you're not just trying to fix a toy but making sure it works the best it can. That's what we want for the person we're looking after.

So, we've learned that when someone has dementia, it's not just their memory that needs help. They need us to be there for them in many ways—like being a good friend who helps when they're sad or being there to laugh with them when they're happy. We also need to make sure they move their bodies, eat foods that are good for them, and do things that make their hearts feel full. This is what we call holistic care.

Remember how we talked about the body's needs? That's like making sure a plant gets water and sunlight. People with dementia need to eat healthy food, move around, and see their doctor to stay as healthy as they can. It's the same with feelings and spirit. They need to feel loved and have peace in their hearts. We can do this by listening to them, sharing stories, and making sure they're not alone too much.

We also learned that being with others is very important. It helps the person with dementia remember how to talk and think, and it keeps their hearts happy. This means doing things like going to a group where they can make friends or having family come over to visit.

Now, you might be wondering how to make all this happen. Well, we talked about that too. Making a care plan is like drawing a map to find treasure. The treasure here is the best care for the person with dementia. This plan looks at what they like, what they need, and how they feel. Then we put it all together in a list that tells us what to do each day.

Let's go over the steps to make this care plan:

- Think about what the person enjoys doing. Maybe they like music or being outside.

- Find out what they need for their body, like what foods are best for them or how much sleep they need.

- Make sure to have time for feelings. This can be quiet time or sharing stories.

- Plan for them to be with others. This could be a game night or a visit to a friend's house.

- Write all these things down in a way that's easy to follow every day.

This chapter was all about making sure we take care of the whole person, not just parts. When we do this, we help them feel their best. And when they feel their best, we feel good too. It's a way to make sure everyone is happy and healthy.

So, take these steps and use them in your care. You'll see how it makes a big difference for the person with dementia and for you. It's a way to show how much you care and want the best for them. And when you need help, remember that you're not alone. There are others out there who want to help you be the best caregiver you can be.

Now that we've gone over everything again, I hope it's clear how important this whole-person approach is. It's something that can really change how we look after someone with dementia. And if you found this helpful, think about joining our community. We have more tips and stories to share. Plus, you can sign up for our newsletter to get the latest updates. There are even courses you can take to learn more about caring for someone with dementia.

Thanks for taking the time to learn about this. It's a big step in making sure you and the person you care for are living the best life you can. Remember, it's all about love, care, and making each day count.

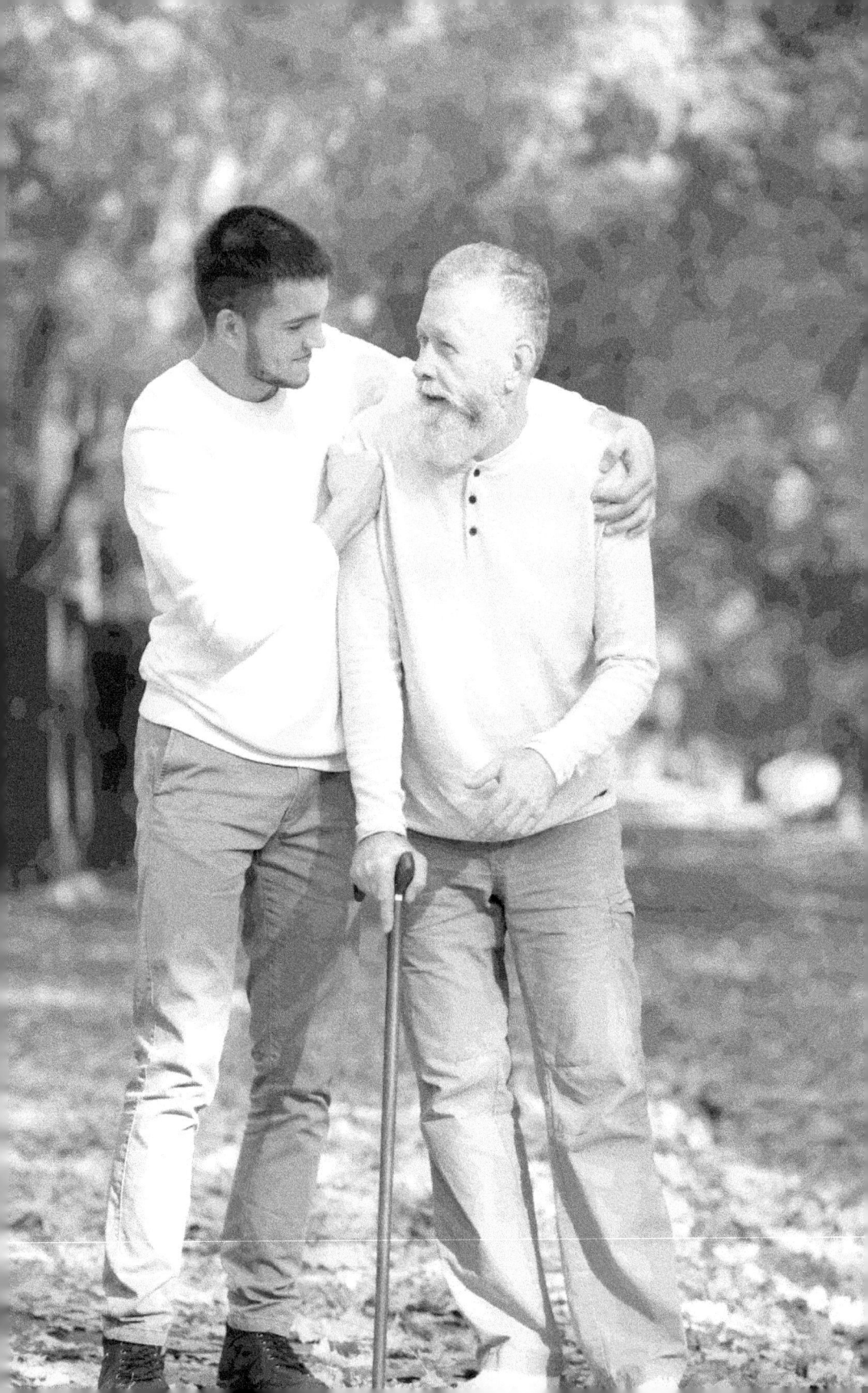

Chapter Eight.
Inspiration for Caregivers

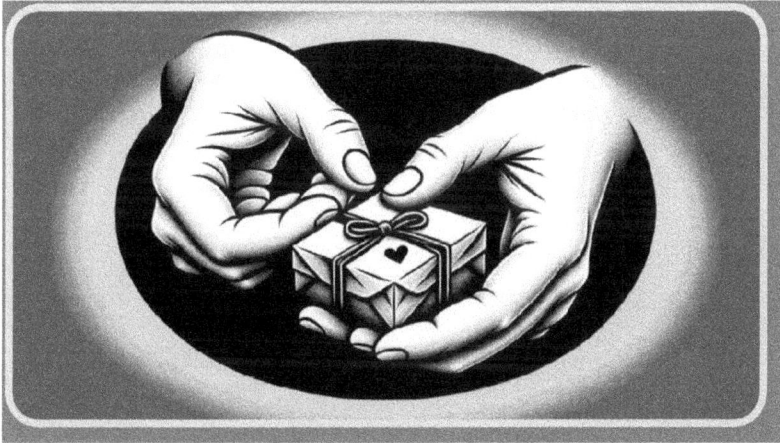

"It's not how much you do, but how much love you put into doing."

– Mother Teresa

Finding Inspiration Amidst Challenges

When you're a caregiver, and some days are tough. You might feel tired or sad. But even on those days, there's something special inside you. It's a little spark. That spark is inspiration. And guess what? It's there to help you through.

Now, you might be wondering, *What is inspiration?* It's a feeling that makes you want to do things. It makes you feel strong and happy. You can find it in different places. You might see a beautiful sunrise and feel ready to start the day. Or maybe you hear a song that makes you want to sing and dance. That's inspiration.

As a caregiver, you help someone every day. You might help them eat or get dressed. Maybe you make them laugh or hold their hand when they're scared. That's a big job. It's hard work. But it's also very, very important. Where do you find your inspiration when things get hard? Let's think about that. Look back at the good days. Think of the smiles and the thank yous. Remember why you started this work. It was because you care. That right there is a source of inspiration. Hold on to that. It's like a light in the dark.

Another place to find inspiration is in the person you're taking care of. They might be fighting a hard battle. Watching them can make you feel strong too. You see their courage, and it lights up that spark inside you. You think, *"If they can do it, so can I."*

It's not just the big things that inspire us. Little things matter too. A kind word. A good meal. A joke that makes both of you laugh. These moments are like fuel. They keep you going. They help you get up and do it all over again the next day.

But sometimes, you need more than memories. You need fresh inspiration. So, go out and look for it. Talk to other caregivers. Listen to their stories. They've had hard days too. They've felt tired and sad. But they keep going. Learn from them. They might have ideas that can help you. They might know about a silly game, a new song, or a different way to do a tough task. That can be just what you need to feel that spark again.

There are also groups and clubs for caregivers. Join one if you can. It's good to talk to people who understand. They know how you feel. They can be your cheerleaders. They can tell you, *"Keep going. You're doing great."* And you can do the same for them. Helping each other is a powerful way to find inspiration.

Books and videos can help too. Look for stories about caregiving. You'll find tips and tricks. You'll read about others who have faced challenges just like yours. You'll see how they found their inspiration. And you'll learn how you can find yours too.

Let's talk about something else now. Every day, you make a choice. You decide to care for someone else. That's a very special thing. You give your time and your love. You make someone's life better. That choice is a big deal. It's something to be proud of. And it's something that can inspire you every single day.

Do you know what else is inspiring? You. Yes, you. You are doing something amazing. Every day, you show up. You do a job that not everyone can do. You make a difference. That's something to celebrate. So, give yourself a pat on the back. You deserve it.

Being a caregiver is a journey. It's not always easy. But remember, you're not alone. There's a whole world of inspiration out there, just waiting for you. And when you find it, you'll feel that spark. It'll warm you up and light the way. So, keep looking for it. Keep talking to others. Keep reading and learning. Keep remembering why you're here. And keep being the wonderful caregiver you are.

That inspiration will help you keep going. It will help you on the days when you're not sure you can do it. It will help you remember that you can. And that you will. Because you're strong. You're caring. And you're inspired.

So, take a deep breath. Let it out. And let's do this. Together. With that spark of inspiration to guide us.

Stories of Resilience and Love

There are stories all around us. Stories that speak of the toughness of the human spirit and the warmth of the human heart. These tales are not just meant to be heard; they're meant to be felt and lived through. They can be a guiding light on a caregiver's path, a path that sometimes feels too rocky, too steep, and too long.

When you care for someone, your days might blend into nights, and the weight of your responsibilities can feel heavy. In these moments, it's stories of resilience and love that can make all the difference. They remind us that we are not alone and that what we do has a lasting impact, not just on the lives of those we care for, but on our own lives too.

Think about a caregiver who has been through what you're going through. What stories might they tell? They might share about the hard days, the ones where nothing seemed to go right. They would tell you about the patience they found deep within, the patience they didn't know they had. The days they kept going, even when they wanted to give up. They might smile as they recall the breakthrough moments, the small victories that felt like winning a war. This is the power of their story— to show you that it's possible to keep moving forward, even when the path is unclear.

Now, what about love? Love is the force that drives every caregiver to do the impossible. The love story of caregiving is not always told with grand gestures. It's in the small, everyday actions. The gentle touch to calm a worried brow. The extra minute spent listening to a story told a hundred times. Love shows up in the warm meal prepared with care and the quiet company in a room filled with silence. It's the love that says, *"You're not alone; I'm here with you."*

These stories of other caregivers are not just tales to be told. They are invitations to you. Invitations to remember why you started this journey. They encourage you to share your own experiences, your own struggles, and your own triumphs. Your story is as powerful as any other. By telling it, you join a community of warriors, each with their own battles, each with their own scars, and each with their own stories of resilience and love.

Sharing your story is not just about finding common ground with others. It's about building a bridge—building understanding, empathy, and connection. When you share, you give a piece of your heart to someone else, and in return, you receive strength. You might not see it right away, but in the sharing, there's healing. In the sharing, there's inspiration.

Let's take a moment to talk about why your story matters. Your story is a beacon of hope for those who feel lost in the dark. It shows them the way. It tells them that despite the challenges, the tears, and the tiredness, there is beauty in caring for another human being. There is a purpose that goes beyond the daily tasks. Your story can shine a light on that purpose, making it clearer and brighter for someone else.

So, how do you begin to tell your story? It starts with a moment, a feeling, a memory. It might start with a challenge you faced head-on. Or perhaps it starts with a moment of unexpected joy amidst a hard day. Begin where you feel the most emotion, because that's where the heart of your story lies. Write it down, speak it out, share it however you can. You never know who needs to hear it, who it might help, or who it might inspire to keep going.

Remember, your story does not need to be perfect. It does not need to be dramatic or filled with heroic acts. Your story is perfect in its truth, in its authenticity. It speaks of your unique journey, your personal battles, and your individual love. That's what makes it powerful. That's what makes it inspiring.

As you move forward in your role as a caregiver, hold on to these stories of resilience and love. Let them be your companions on the days when the road is tough. Let them remind you of the strength that lies within you and the love that guides you. And when you're ready, add your voice to the chorus of stories. Share your experiences. Build that bridge. Find inspiration in your journey, and be the inspiration for someone else's.

Stories have a way of staying with us. They wrap around us like a warm blanket on a cold night. They're a reminder of what's possible. The stories of resilience and love in caregiving are no different. They are powerful. They are transformative. They tell us that no matter what comes our way, we can be tough, and we can be tender. We can face the challenges, and we can do it with love. These stories are not just stories. They are life. They are love. They are us.

So, let's keep these stories close. Let's tell them often. Let's live them even more. And through it all, let's never forget the incredible impact we have as caregivers. Your story is valuable, your care is essential, and your love is transformative. Share it all. It matters more than you might ever know.

Learning from Others

Let's pause for a moment and think about the many people who have walked the path of caregiving before us. It's a journey that can be tough, yes, but it's also filled with stories of hope, courage, and wisdom. These stories aren't just tales to be heard; they're lessons to be learned. So, let's dive into why it's so vital to learn from other caregivers and how this can spark inspiration in our own lives.

Firstly, consider the importance of connection. You see, when we come together as a community of caregivers, we create a network of support that's invaluable. And in this community, there's nothing more heartwarming than hearing about someone who faced similar challenges and triumphed. Hearing a fellow caregiver's success story can be a ray of light on a cloudy day. It reminds us that we are not alone, and that together, we can overcome anything that comes our way.

Now, let's talk about the real, gritty experiences of caregiving. It's not just about success; it's also about the struggles, the late nights, and the early mornings. Sharing these moments with each other helps us understand that it's okay to feel overwhelmed sometimes. We learn that every caregiver has moments of doubt and that it's perfectly normal. Recognizing this can lift a weight off our shoulders, making us feel lighter, and more hopeful.

But how do we use these stories and experiences? To start, we can look for lessons in every story we hear. If a caregiver shares how they managed to keep calm during a particularly tough situation, we can take notes. What did they do? How did they react? We can take these golden nuggets of wisdom and try them out in our own lives. And when we find something that works for us, we can pass it on to help someone else.

Imagine you're sitting around a table with a group of caregivers, each sharing a piece of their journey. One talks about the joy they found in the small moments, like a smile from the person they care for. Another speaks about the strength they discovered within themselves. As you listen, you find your own spirits lifting. You realize that your role as a caregiver is not just about the tasks you do; it's about the love and the life you bring into the lives of others. This is learning from others at its best.

And what about those days when everything seems to go wrong? When the person you're caring for is having a tough day, and you're exhausted? In our community, we share those days too. We talk about what kept us going, maybe a kind word from a friend or a helpful tip from another caregiver. We learn that it's okay to seek help, to take a moment for ourselves, and to recharge. This is the kind of learning that strengthens us, and prepares us for the days ahead.

It's also about practical advice. Maybe you're trying to find a way to manage your time better, or you're looking for resources to help with caregiving. By talking to others, you can discover how they tackle these issues. Perhaps they have a checklist that could work for you, or they know of a local group that offers the support you need. These are actionable steps that you can put into practice right away. They're small changes, but they can make a big difference in your day-to-day life.

And then, let's not forget about the emotional side of things. Caregiving can tug at your heartstrings. Sharing feelings with others who understand can be incredibly healing. It's a chance to open up, to say, *"This is hard,"* and to hear someone else respond, *"I know, I've been there too."* It's in these shared emotions that we find a common thread, a sense of belonging, and a source of inspiration to keep going.

So, how do we create this community of support? We can start small. It could be as simple as joining a caregiver's group online or attending a local meet-up. The key is to start sharing your own story, and your own insights. You might be surprised at how much you have to offer and how much you'll get in return. It's a beautiful exchange, one that enriches everyone involved.

Lastly, remember this: learning from others is a journey, not a destination. It's a continuous process that evolves as we move forward in our caregiving roles.

Each person we meet, and each story we hear, adds another layer to our understanding and resilience. It's a treasure trove of inspiration that we can dip into whenever we need it.

So here we are, at the end of our conversation for now. Remember, the wisdom of fellow caregivers is a gift—one that keeps on giving. It's there for us to learn from, to draw strength from, and to pass on. Let's embrace this with open hearts and minds. Let's learn from each other and keep the inspiration alive. Because together, we are an unstoppable force of care, love, and hope.

Cultivating Personal Inspiration

When you wake up each morning, what's the first thing that comes to your mind? Maybe it's the list of tasks that lie ahead or the people you care for. Being a caregiver is a role filled with many moments—some are rewarding, and others are tough. But through it all, it's crucial to keep your inner flame of motivation burning brightly. This inner flame is your personal inspiration. It's what gets you through the day, no matter how challenging it may be. So, how do you keep this flame alive? Let's talk about that.

Personal inspiration is like the fuel for your car. Without it, you can't move forward. Think of the last time you felt truly inspired. What was it that sparked that feeling? Maybe it was a kind word from someone you helped or a small victory you achieved. These sparks are everywhere, but you need to recognize them and use them to light your fire.

Let's start with the basics. You need to know what inspires you. This is not always as easy as it sounds. You may need to sit down and think hard about what brings you joy, hope, and energy. It could be something big, like the dream of a future goal, or something small, like the smile on a loved one's face.

Once you've figured out what your sources of inspiration are, it's time to turn them into a daily ritual. A personal ritual or practice doesn't have to be complicated. It can be as simple as reading a motivational quote every morning or taking a few minutes to enjoy a cup of tea in silence. What matters is that it helps you connect with that inspiration every single day.

Why is this important? Because caregiving is not a one-day event. It's a journey that you're on, and like any long journey, there will be times when you feel like you can't take another step. That's when your personal inspiration ritual becomes a lifeline. It's the steady beat of a drum that keeps you marching forward. It's the warmth of the sun on your back, even on a cold day.

Now you might wonder, *what if you don't feel inspired?* What if, despite your best efforts, the flame just doesn't seem to ignite? This is where you need to be a bit of a detective. You see, inspiration isn't just about feeling good. It's about understanding what drives you and using that knowledge to push through the tough times.

Let's say you love reading stories about other caregivers. These stories make you feel like you're not alone. They make you feel connected to a larger community of people who understand what you're going through. So make it a practice to read these stories regularly. Find books, blogs, or forums where these stories are shared. Allow the experiences of others to fuel your own journey.

But let's be clear, cultivating personal inspiration is not about ignoring the hard parts of caregiving. It's about finding a balance. It's about giving yourself the strength to face the difficult moments with the same grace and courage as you do the happy ones.

To maintain this balance, it's helpful to have a variety of inspiration sources. Think of it as having a toolbox. In this toolbox, you have different tools for different situations. A kind word here, a success story there, perhaps a treasured memory or a future dream. You can reach into this toolbox whenever you need a little boost.

Don't underestimate the power of small, everyday joys. The laughter of a friend, the beauty of a sunrise, the satisfaction of a job well done. These small sparks can become big flames if you let them. They can light up the dark corners of your day and remind you of why you do what you do.

Another important aspect is to share your inspiration. Talk about what inspires you with the people you care for. You might discover that your sources of inspiration are contagious. When you share your passion, it can ignite a similar passion in others. This creates a positive feedback loop that not only keeps you inspired but also spreads that inspiration to those around you.

Additionally, remember to be kind to yourself. There will be days when even the strongest sources of inspiration don't seem to work. On those days, it's okay to just *be*. To take a step back and rest. To recharge your batteries so that you can come back stronger tomorrow. Inspiration is not a sprint; it's a marathon.

And when you do find yourself feeling inspired, take a moment to savor it. Let that feeling sink in. Remember what it feels like, so you can recall it when you need it the most. Write it down, take a photo, and do whatever you need to do to capture that moment of inspiration.

In the end, cultivating personal inspiration is about understanding yourself as much as it is about caring for others. It's about creating a space where you can tap into the things that give you strength and joy. It's a journey within a journey, and it's one of the most important ones you'll ever take.

So, dear caregiver, take the time to cultivate your personal inspiration. Make it a part of your daily life. Use it to fuel your passion for caregiving. And remember, you're not just helping others; you're also building a life filled with purpose and meaning for yourself.

Now, as you continue with your day, think about what inspires you. Think about how you can turn that inspiration into a daily practice. And if you're struggling to find your spark, reach out. Talk to friends, family, or fellow caregivers. Look for inspiration in books, music, art, or nature. Remember, you're not alone on this journey. Together, we can keep the flame of inspiration burning brightly in all of our hearts.

Overcoming Inspirational Roadblocks

When we care for others, sometimes we hit a wall. It's like finding a big rock in the middle of our path. It's hard, and it can make us feel like we can't keep going. But here's the thing: we can get past that big rock. We can keep moving forward with the right steps. I'm here to talk about those steps.

First, let's think about what makes us feel stuck. Sometimes, we feel tired. We may feel like no one sees what we're doing. Or we might think that what we do is not making a difference. These thoughts can be big roadblocks to feeling good about our work as caregivers. But they don't have to stop us.

One thing we can do is remind ourselves why we started. Why did we want to help in the first place? Most of us started because we care. We care a lot. Remembering that can be a bright light on a dark day. It can help us push the big rock out of the way.

Then, there's talking to someone. When things get hard, we should find someone to talk to. It could be a friend or someone else who knows about caring for people. They can help us see that we're not alone. This can make our hearts feel a little lighter. And when our hearts feel lighter, that big rock starts to feel smaller.

Writing things down can help too. We can take a little notebook and write what we feel. We can write the good things and the not-so-good things. This can help us see what's really making us feel stuck. It's like a map that shows us where the big rock is. Once we see it, we can start to move it out of the way.

Sometimes, we also need to take a break. That's okay. It's like sitting down to rest when we've been walking for a long time. When we rest, we get our strength back. Then, we can stand up and start moving past that big rock again.

Also, let's think about the people we care for. They smile. They say thank you. They count on us. These are the little things that can make a big difference. They are like a soft wind that helps push the big rock away.

It's important to look back, too. Look at all the days we've helped others. We've done a lot! That shows how strong we are. Even when that big rock seems to be in the way, we've still moved forward a lot. And we can keep on going.

There's something else we can do. We can learn new things. Learning makes us smarter and stronger. When we learn, we find new tools to help us move that big rock. And with those new tools, the job gets a little easier.

What if we try to see things in a new way? Maybe the big rock in the path is not really stopping us. Maybe it's just making us slow down for a bit. That's not always bad. It can give us time to think and to find new ways around the rock.

Here is one more idea. Let's celebrate the small wins. Every little step we take is a win. When we look at all those little wins, they add up to something big. They show us that we are moving the rock, even when it feels like we're not. Remember, we do an important job. We help people. We make their days better. Even on days when that big rock seems to be in our way, we are doing something that really matters.

We can get past the roadblocks. We can keep doing our work with love and care. We can keep helping those who need us. And we can do it with a full heart, knowing that every day, we make the world a little better.

So, to you, the caregiver who feels the weight of the rock, know this: you are not alone. You are strong. And together, we can move mountains, one small rock at a time.

Recap: Inspired Caregiving

Let's talk about inspiration. It's like the air we breathe. It's all around us, even when we're caring for someone else. Sometimes, it's easy to find. Other times, it's like a game of hide and seek. But as a caregiver, you need it. Oh, you need it so much. It's what keeps you going when the days are long and tough.

So, where do you find this inspiration? Remember, it's as much within you as it is outside. Take a step back and look. See the smile of the person you care for? That's inspiration. How about when they manage to do something new, something they couldn't do before? That's a big win. That's inspiration right there.

But I know what you're thinking. It's not always that simple. Inspiration can slip away on hard days. So here's the secret: You've got to keep it close, hold onto it tight. You're doing important work. Very important work. You're a giver of care, of love, of life. That's something to be proud of.

Now, let's dig in. How do you keep that inspiration alive, day after day? First, create a ritual. It could be reading a story, taking a walk, or just spending a few quiet moments with your thoughts. This ritual is your anchor. It's what you'll turn to when you need to remind yourself why you do what you do.

Next, connect with others. Yes, others like you. There's a whole world of caregivers out there. They have stories that will lift you up, make you laugh, and fill you with hope. Speak to them. Listen to them. Share your story too. It's a two-way street, this sharing of inspiration.

But what happens when you hit a roadblock? It's okay. It happens to everyone. The trick is to not let it stay. Look that challenge in the eye and say, *"Not today."* You've got tools to get past it. Focus on the good you're doing. The love you're sharing. The lives you're touching.

Don't forget to take care of yourself, too. Self-care isn't selfish. It's essential. When you're feeling good, you can give good. And that's what this is all about, right?

Now, here's what you can do today, and every day, to keep that spark of inspiration glowing:

• Start a gratitude journal. Every night, write down three things that made you feel inspired that day.

• Create a vision board. Fill it with pictures and words that reflect your hopes and dreams as a caregiver.

• Set a daily reminder on your phone. Have it pop up with a positive message or a goal for the day.

• Find a caregiving buddy. Someone to talk to when you need a boost or a shoulder to lean on.

• Learn something new about caregiving. Knowledge is power, and it's also inspiring.

• Give yourself a break. When it's time to rest, rest. You'll come back stronger.

• Do something that makes you happy. Dance, sing, paint, run. Do what lights you up inside.

See, these steps are simple. But they're powerful. They're doable. You can start them today. And they will make a difference. A big difference. What you do matters. It matters so much. You might not always see it, but you're making the world a better place, one act of care at a time. Hold onto that. That's your flame of inspiration. And it's burning bright.

Stick with these steps. They're your map to staying inspired. And when you're inspired, you inspire others. It's like a chain of goodness that just keeps going. And that, my friend, is a beautiful thing.

You're not alone. Remember that. You're part of a community, a family of caregivers. Together, we hold onto inspiration. Together, we keep moving forward. Because that's what caregivers do. We care, we love, and we inspire. So, take a deep breath. You've got this. You really do. And when you wake up tomorrow, know that you're stepping into a day full of possibilities. A day where you can be the inspiration you're looking for.

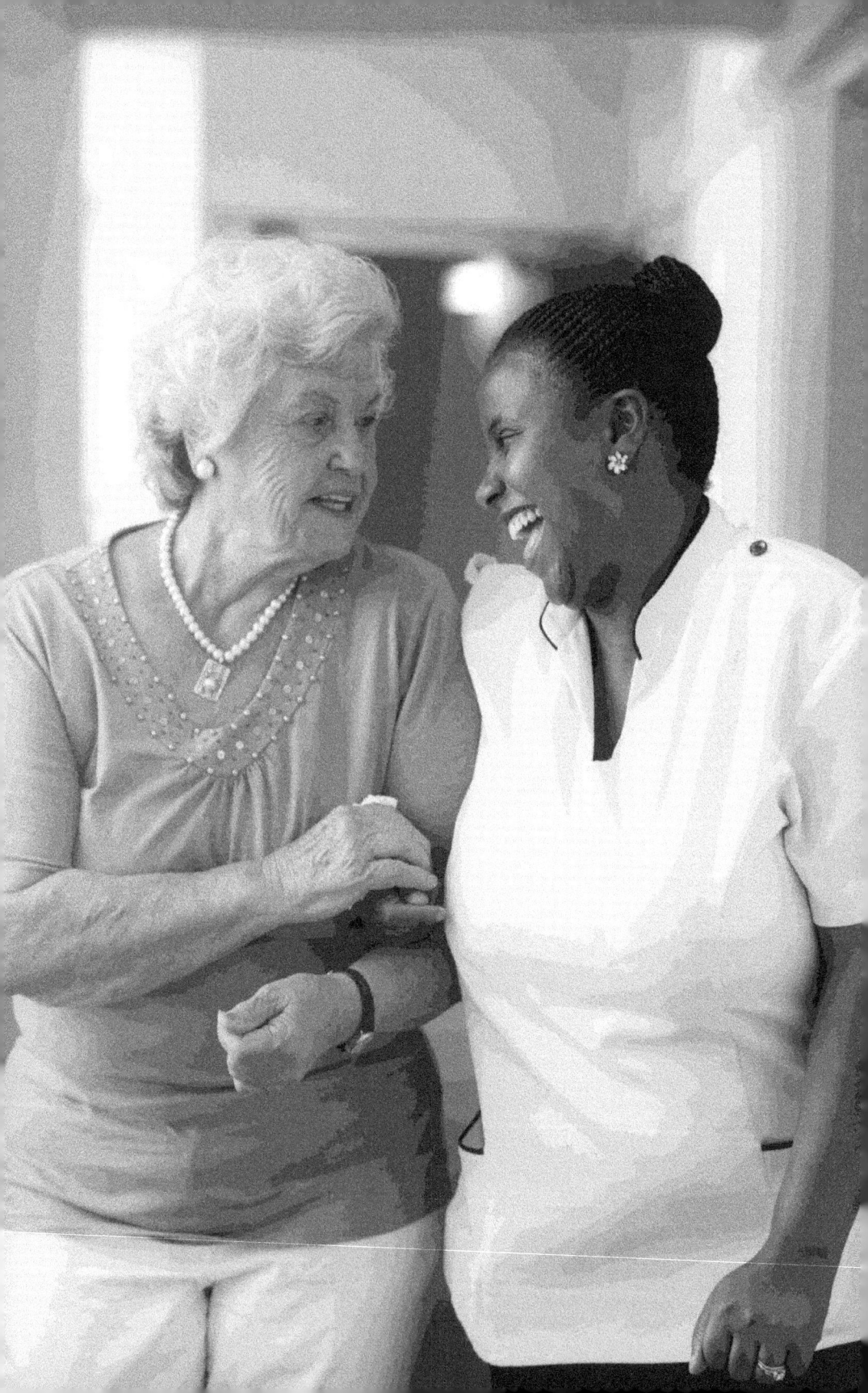

Chapter Nine.
Zeal for Caregiving

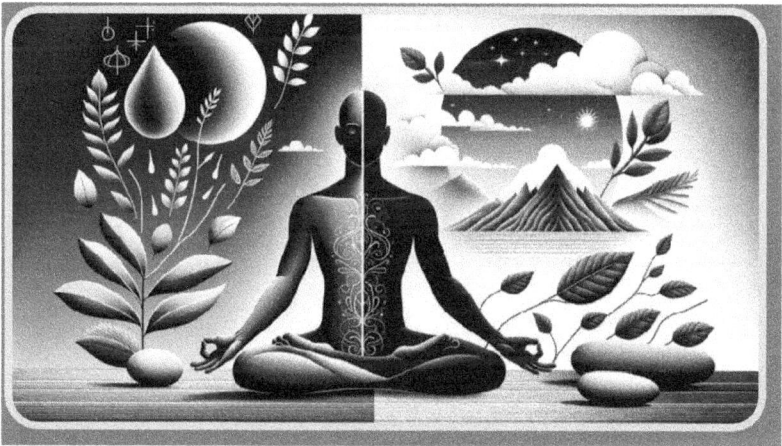

"Taking time to meditate is as important as taking the time to breathe. One pumps oxygen into the body, the other pumps peace into the mind."

– Marianne Williamson

Cultivating Zeal through Spiritual Healing

Taking care of someone is a big job. It takes a lot of time and love. If you're a caregiver, you know how hard it can be. Some days, you might feel really tired. You might even feel like you're doing the same things over and over. But here's something special: there's a way to bring back your energy and joy. It's called **spiritual healing**. This can help you feel strong and happy again. Spiritual healing is when you use your heart and spirit to feel better. It's not just about your body; it's about your feelings and your peace of mind.

When you take care of your heart and spirit, you can take care of others better too. Let's talk about how we can do this. **Meditation** is one way to heal your spirit. It's when you sit quietly and let your thoughts go. You try to think about nothing or focus on something simple, like your breathing. This helps your mind stop racing.

When you meditate, you can find a calm place inside you. This calm place can help you through tough days.

Another part of spiritual healing is **breathing exercises**. Breathing is something we all do, but did you know that the way you breathe can change how you feel? There are special ways to breathe that can make you feel more awake and alive. These exercises are simple. You can do them anytime, anywhere. Let's try one together.

Sit in a chair or on the floor. Sit up straight. Now, breathe in slowly through your nose. Fill your lungs with air. Hold it for just a moment. Then, let it out slowly through your mouth. Do this a few times. Can you feel a difference? It's like giving your body a mini-nap. After that, you might feel like you can think better and have more energy.

And here's why this is important: When you feel good, you can do a better job taking care of others. If you're happy and full of energy, the person you're taking care of can feel that too. It makes them feel better. Your good feelings can spread to them. It's like sharing a smile. One person smiles, then another person smiles back. It's the same with feeling calm and happy.

Taking care of your spirit also means doing things that make your heart happy. Maybe you like music. You can sing or listen to your favorite songs. Or maybe you like to draw or paint. Doing things you enjoy is good for your spirit. It's important to make time for these things, even when you're busy.

When you're a caregiver, you give a lot of yourself. You help someone with their needs, but you have needs too. Your heart and spirit need care. When you take care of your spirit, you can keep giving to others. You can keep your joy. And that's a beautiful thing.

Let's remember this: Caring for others is a big job, but caring for yourself is just as important. When you feel good, you can help others feel good too. We all need help sometimes, and we all need to feel loved. You're doing a great job as a caregiver. And with spiritual healing, you can feel even better. So, keep doing your breathing exercises. Keep finding time to meditate. Do things that make you happy. This is how you keep your zeal. This is how you take the best care of others and yourself. It's a wonderful thing you're doing. Keep up the great work. And remember, taking care of your spirit means taking care of everything.

Rediscovering Joy in Caregiving through Mindfulness and Meditation

So, let's talk about joy. Yes, joy. This simple word can bring a smile to your face, right? Now, think about caregiving. It's hard work. But what if I told you that you can find joy in caregiving too? It's true, and I'll tell you how. **Mindfulness** and **meditation** can help you find that joy, even in tough times.

Mindfulness is about being in the moment. It's like when you are watching a beautiful sunset. You are not thinking about yesterday or tomorrow. Just the colors and the peace of that moment. When you are giving care to someone, being in the moment helps you focus on the care you give. It makes the care better for you and the person you are helping.

Now, let's add meditation. Meditation is sitting quietly and letting your thoughts come and go. It is like when you sit by a river and watch the water flow by.

223

Thoughts are like the water. They come, and they go. When you meditate, you learn to not hold on to these thoughts. You just let them flow. This helps your mind feel clear and calm.

Why are mindfulness and meditation important in caregiving? Well, sometimes caregiving can feel like too much. It can make you tired and stressed. But when you practice being mindful, you can see caregiving in a new way. You can see the smiles, the thankfulness, and the little moments that make it all worth it. Being mindful helps you remember why you started caregiving in the first place. It was not just a job, right? It was because you care. Meditation helps you keep your mind strong, so you can keep caring, even when it's hard.

Here's how you can start being more mindful today. First, find a quiet place. It can be anywhere that feels calm to you. Sit or stand there. Now, take a deep breath in and let it out slowly. Do this a few times. Feel your feet on the ground. Listen to the sounds around you.

What do you hear? What do you feel? This is you being in the moment. This is mindfulness.

If you want to try meditation, it's just as simple. Find your quiet place again. Sit down this time. Close your eyes if you want. Now breathe in and out slowly. When thoughts come into your mind, it's okay. Just let them go like the water in the river. Start with just a few minutes each day. You can meditate longer when you feel ready.

Why should you do all this? Well, when you are mindful and when you meditate, you can handle stress better. You can find joy in the little things. And when you find joy, the person you are caring for can feel it too. It's like when someone smiles at you, and you can't help but smile back. Joy is catchy like that.

So, caregivers, this is for you. When days are long and hard, remember to take a moment for yourself. Be mindful. Meditate. Find the joy in the work you do. You are not just doing a job; you are making a difference in someone's life. And that, my friends, is something to find joy in every day.

But wait, there's more you can do. When you go to work tomorrow, try this. As you start each task, take a moment. Think about what you are doing and why. Are you making someone comfortable? Are you helping someone eat a tasty meal? These are good things. Be proud of them. Feel the joy in these moments.

Again, you are not alone. All caregivers can share in this joy. Talk to each other. Share your mindfulness tips. Share what makes you happy in your work. When one caregiver is happy, it can spread to others. It's like when one person starts clapping, and soon everyone is clapping. Joy can spread that way too.

To wrap it up, being a caregiver is important. It's not always easy, but there's joy in it. Mindfulness and meditation can help you find that joy. They can help you stay calm and strong. And when you are calm and strong, you can give the best care. You can make every day a little better for you and for the person you care for.

Start small. A few minutes of mindfulness or meditation are all it takes to begin. Each day, you can grow this practice. Soon, you'll find that joy in caregiving you may have thought was lost. It's there, waiting for you. Just take a breath, be in the moment, and let the joy of caring shine through.

Breathing Exercises for Overcoming Monotony

When you care for someone every day, you might feel like you're doing the same things over and over. It's like when you hear the same song too many times—it can get boring. But here's the thing: a simple act of breathing in a new way can make a big difference. Yes, it's about breathing exercises that can help you feel less bored and more alive. Now, let me walk you through these steps and explain why each one matters.

Breathing is something we all do without thinking, but when you focus on it, it becomes a powerful tool. You see, breathing exercises can help you feel calm and bring new energy to your body. It's something you can do anytime, anywhere, and it doesn't cost a thing.

The first thing to do is find a quiet spot. This can be anywhere you feel safe and can relax for a few minutes. Once you're there, sit down or stand still. Let your body be comfortable. Now, close your eyes if you like. This helps you focus on your breath and nothing else.

Next, take a deep breath in through your nose. Let the air fill your lungs slowly, all the way down to your belly. Think of it like filling a cup with water, from the bottom to the top. Hold that breath for just a moment. Then, let it out through your mouth, nice and slow. As you breathe out, imagine all the boredom and tiredness leaving your body with the air. It's like letting go of a balloon and watching it fly away.

Do this by breathing in and out a few times. Keep it slow and steady. Each time you breathe in, think about fresh energy coming into your body. And each time you breathe out, think about the dull feelings going away. It's a simple thing, but it can make you feel so much better.

Now, let's add a little counting to the mix. When you breathe in, count to four in your head: one, two, three, four. Hold your breath for another count of four. Then, breathe out for four counts. Doing this counting can help your mind stay on track. It's like following the steps in a dance, and it keeps your thoughts from wandering off.

After you've done this for a few minutes, you'll probably start to notice a change. Your body might feel lighter, and your mind might feel clearer. This is your body saying thank you for giving it a little break and some fresh air. It's a simple trick, but it can make the rest of your day feel a little brighter. Remember, you can do this any time you start to feel the boredom creeping in. Whether you're waiting for something, or you've just finished a task, take a few minutes to breathe like this. It's a handy tool you can use all day long.

But wait, there's more you can do with your breath. Try breathing in for four counts, holding for seven counts, and breathing out for eight counts. This is a bit longer and can take a bit of practice. But it's a great way to give your brain and body a big reset button.

Here's one more tip. If you're feeling really stuck, stand up and stretch your arms high while you breathe in. Then, as you breathe out, let your arms fall slowly to your sides. Do this a few times. It's like you're reaching for new energy and then wrapping it around you.

These breathing exercises are something you can share, too. If you know someone else who feels the same way you do, show them how to do this. It's a nice way to help each other out. And doing it together can make it even more fun.

So, that's how you can use breathing to help you when things feel too similar. Remember to do these exercises often. They can help you feel more awake, more alive, and ready to enjoy caring for others again. Plus, when you breathe better, you feel better, and that's good for everyone around you, too.

Before we finish, let's make sure you've got everything you need. You know to find a quiet place. You know to breathe in slowly and fill your lungs. You know to hold that breath and then let it out gently. You know about counting to keep your mind focused. And you know you can stretch and move to make it even better. These are the steps to make breathing exercises

231

work for you. And don't forget, when you feel good, the person you're caring for can feel it, too. They might not say it, but they can sense it. Your good mood and energy can make their day brighter as well.

So, there you go. You've got a new tool in your caregiving toolbox. Use it as much as you like. It's free, it's easy, and it's all yours. And who knows? It might just turn a boring day into a better one. Breathe well, feel good, and keep on caring with a happy heart. That's what it's all about.

Spiritual Practices for Energizing Self and Others

When we give care to others, especially in demanding roles like caregiving for individuals with dementia, it's easy to feel like our inner light dims a bit. Day in, and day out, we focus on the needs of someone else, and this can sometimes leave us feeling a little less bright ourselves. But there's good news. There's something that can help us glow again, and even better, it can help everyone we work with shine too. It's called **spiritual practice**, and it's not as complex as it might sound.

Spiritual practices are like food for our souls. They feed us with motivation and fill us with energy. You don't have to believe in anything specific or belong to any particular group to enjoy these practices. They are for everyone, no matter what you think about the world. They are simple actions or thoughts that make us feel connected to something bigger. They make us feel alive, fresh, and full of zest—ready to take on the world.

One of the simplest ways to start is with something we all do every day—**breathing**. But this is not just any breath. This is a deep, purposeful breath. When you breathe in, imagine you are pulling in positive energy from around you. And when you breathe out, picture sending out all the tiredness and stress. This can be done anywhere and anytime. You don't need any special tools or a quiet room. Just a few minutes and your breath.

Let's add a little twist to it. Let's get together with others. Yes, you heard that right. Find your fellow caregivers and breathe together. You can stand in a circle, sit around a table, or even do it virtually over a call. When you breathe in sync with others, there's a sense of unity that comes alive. It's as if you're not just sharing a space but also sharing strength, courage, and motivation. And that feeling can power you through even the toughest days.

Now let's talk about a different kind of practice. It's called **gratitude**. Every day, think of three things you are grateful for. They could be small, like a delicious cup of coffee, or big, like the love of a family member. Share these with your team. Let them share theirs with you. When we focus on what we're thankful for, it's like flipping a switch in our minds. We move from thinking about what we don't have to appreciate what we do. This can transform our mood and our whole approach to caregiving.

Here's another idea. Set up a little corner in your workspace for peace. You can call it the peace corner, the zen zone, or anything that feels right. Put up pictures, quotes, or anything else that brings you a sense of calm. Invite your colleagues to add to it. This place can become a shared sanctuary, a spot where anyone can go for a quick moment of rest and recharge. When you've got a peaceful spot to rest your eyes, even just for a few seconds, it's astonishing how much more energized you can feel.

Finally, let's not forget the power of a shared smile or a kind word. It costs nothing to tell someone they're doing great. It takes no time to give a simple compliment. These are tiny acts of spiritual practice, and they work wonders. When we lift each other up, the whole team rises. When one person shines, it's easier for us all to sparkle just a bit more.

In conclusion, spiritual practices don't have to be grand or complicated. They're about finding simple ways to connect, to fill our hearts with joy, and to spread that energy to others. When we practice together, the bond between us grows stronger, and our capacity to care becomes greater. So breathe deeply, share gratitude, create peaceful spaces, and remember the power of kindness. These small, simple actions can reignite the passion and enthusiasm needed for a fulfilling caregiving journey. By energizing ourselves and our fellow caregivers, we not only improve our own well-being but also enhance the care and compassion we provide to those who rely on us.

Promoting a Positive Outlook through Spiritual Connection

What does it mean to have a **positive outlook**? It's the way you see things around you, the way you think about the people you care for, and the kind of vibe you give off. This isn't just about feeling good; it's about creating a space where you and the people you look after can feel at ease, happy, and peaceful. Let's talk about how you can make this happen with something special called a **spiritual connection**. It's quite a beautiful thing, really.

First, let's think about spiritual connection. This isn't about religion or belief in something specific. It's about connecting to something bigger than ourselves. It might be love, nature, or the feeling you get when you help someone. It's that heartwarming sensation that swells inside you and spreads all around. This kind of connection can make a huge difference in caregiving.

It starts with you, the caregiver. When you tap into this sense of connection, it's like you're filling your heart with sunshine. That warmth doesn't stay just in your heart. Oh no, it spreads. It touches everyone around you, especially the person you're caring for. Imagine a smile that lights up a room. That's what we're talking about here. The power of your outlook can change the whole mood of where you are and what you're doing.

How do you make this spiritual connection? You might be thinking, "That sounds hard." But it's not. It's all about finding moments in your day to pause, breathe, and feel the goodness inside you.

Take a deep breath right now. Go on, a really deep one. Let it out slowly. There you go. At that moment, you were connected. Do this often, and you'll start to feel that positive vibe grow. It's like watering a plant. Give it what it needs, and watch it flourish.

Let's be real: Caregiving is tough. Some days, it can feel like you're climbing a mountain that never ends. But here's a secret: Your spiritual connection is like a pair of super-powered hiking boots. It helps you keep going with a bounce in your step. It gives you strength. And when you reach out with a heart full of this power, it helps the person you're caring for feel stronger too. They can sense your calm, your hope, and your joy. It's contagious in the best kind of way.

You might wonder, "What if I don't feel that connection every day?" That's okay. We're all humans. Some days the connection will feel strong, and other days, you might need to look for it a little harder. But don't give up. Keep looking for those moments to connect.

Listen to your favorite song, watch a sunrise, or share a laugh. These are the things that recharge your spirit. And when your spirit is charged, it shines. You become a lighthouse in the fog for those you're helping.

This isn't about doing anything big or fancy. It's about simple things. It's about being present in the moment and finding joy in small acts of kindness. When you hand someone a cup of tea, do it with love. When you listen, really listen. It's in these simple acts that you'll find that glowing thread of spiritual connection. You'll be surprised at how much it can change things for the better.

Now, how can you make sure you keep this connection strong? **Practice**, my friend. Practice. Just like playing an instrument or learning to read, the more you do it, the better you get. Spend some time each day in quiet reflection. Maybe when you wake up or before you sleep. Think about the good you've done, the smiles you've shared, and the love you've felt. Let those feelings fill you up. It's like saving up sunshine for a rainy day.

And guess what? This positive outlook you're creating is good for your health too. When you're happy and at peace, your body feels it. It's like giving your body a big, cozy hug from the inside. So, you're not just helping the person you care for; you're helping yourself too. It's a win-win!

One last thing. Don't keep this secret to yourself. Share it with other caregivers. Talk about the good things, the tough things, and how you find your connection. The more you share, the more you'll find that others are on this journey with you. Together, you'll create a circle of positivity that can hold up even on the hardest days.

So, to wrap this up, remember that promoting a positive outlook through spiritual connection is all about the little things. The deep breaths, the quiet moments of reflection, and the simple acts of kindness. These are the building blocks of a joyful caregiving experience. Keep practicing, keep sharing, and watch as you, those you care for, and those you work with start to glow with that inner sunshine. It's amazing what a difference it can make.

And before I forget, if you ever want to learn more about this or anything else to do with caregiving, we've got tons of resources. Consider joining our community, subscribing to our newsletter, or taking our courses.

We've got your back, and we're here to help you shine. Take care, keep connecting, and let that positive outlook light up the world around you.

Recap: Embracing Spiritual Practices for Sustained Zeal

We just explored some wonderful ways to bring back that spark in caregiving. Caregiving is not just a task; it's more than that. It's a journey, a path that intertwines with another person's life. But, like any journey, it can sometimes feel long and tiring. Don't worry. We're here to help each other keep that inner flame alive. So let's talk about how to keep your fire burning bright.

Spiritual healing is powerful. It helps us stay strong and committed. When we talk about meditation and breathing exercises, we're talking about tools that help your mind and emotions feel better. Imagine feeling calm and at peace every day. This can be your reality if you include these practices in your day. Now, mindfulness and meditation may sound big, but they're really simple.

When you're doing small tasks, like making a bed or preparing a meal, you can be **mindful**. This means you pay attention to what you're doing. You notice how the sheets feel or how the food smells. It's like watching a movie and focusing only on that, nothing else. This helps you find joy in the little things.

But how about when things get dull? **Breathing exercises** are like a fresh breeze on a warm day. They can wake up your mind and body. If you feel stuck in the same old routine, try taking a deep breath in, hold it, and then let it out slowly. Do this a few times. Feel better? That's the magic of breathing.

We can share this magic with others, too. When we do these exercises with our fellow caregivers, we make a team that's full of energy and support. It's like when birds fly together; they go further. And we want to go further in our caregiving, don't we?

Now, let's not forget about being positive. When we **connect with something bigger than us**, it's easier to see the good in life. This doesn't mean everything is perfect, but it means we can handle things better. We can be peaceful and kind, even when tough times come our way. And this helps everyone, not just us, but also the people we care for.

So, how do you start with all this? It's simple:

- **Set aside a little time each day for yourself.** This is your time to do a bit of meditation or breathing. Find a quiet spot. Sit or stand comfortably. Close your eyes. Breathe deeply. Feel your lungs fill up and then empty out. Do this for a few minutes. It's like giving your mind a short vacation.

- **When you're doing tasks, focus on them.** Notice everything about what you're doing. If your mind wanders, that's okay. Just bring it back. It's like a puppy that runs off. Gently bring it back to where you want it.

- **Chat with others about trying these exercises together.** Maybe before your shifts start, you can all do a quick meditation. It's like stretching before a big game. It gets you ready and feeling good.

- **Remember to think about the good things**. Even on hard days, there's always something good. Find it. Hold onto it. Share it with others. It's like finding a pretty shell on the beach. It makes the whole day better.

These steps are simple but powerful. They help you care for others and yourself. This is important because **you are important**. Your work as a caregiver is a gift. And when you feel good, you give the best of yourself to others. That's a beautiful thing.

Keep these ideas in your heart as you go through your days. They can turn an ordinary day into something special. You have the power to keep that **zeal**, that passion for caregiving, alive and well. And that's a win for everyone. It's a win for you, the person you care for, and the whole caregiving community. And remember, you're never alone in this. We're all on this journey together.

Let's keep walking this path with joy and with that fire in our hearts. That's the key to being the best caregivers we can be. **Let's do this!**

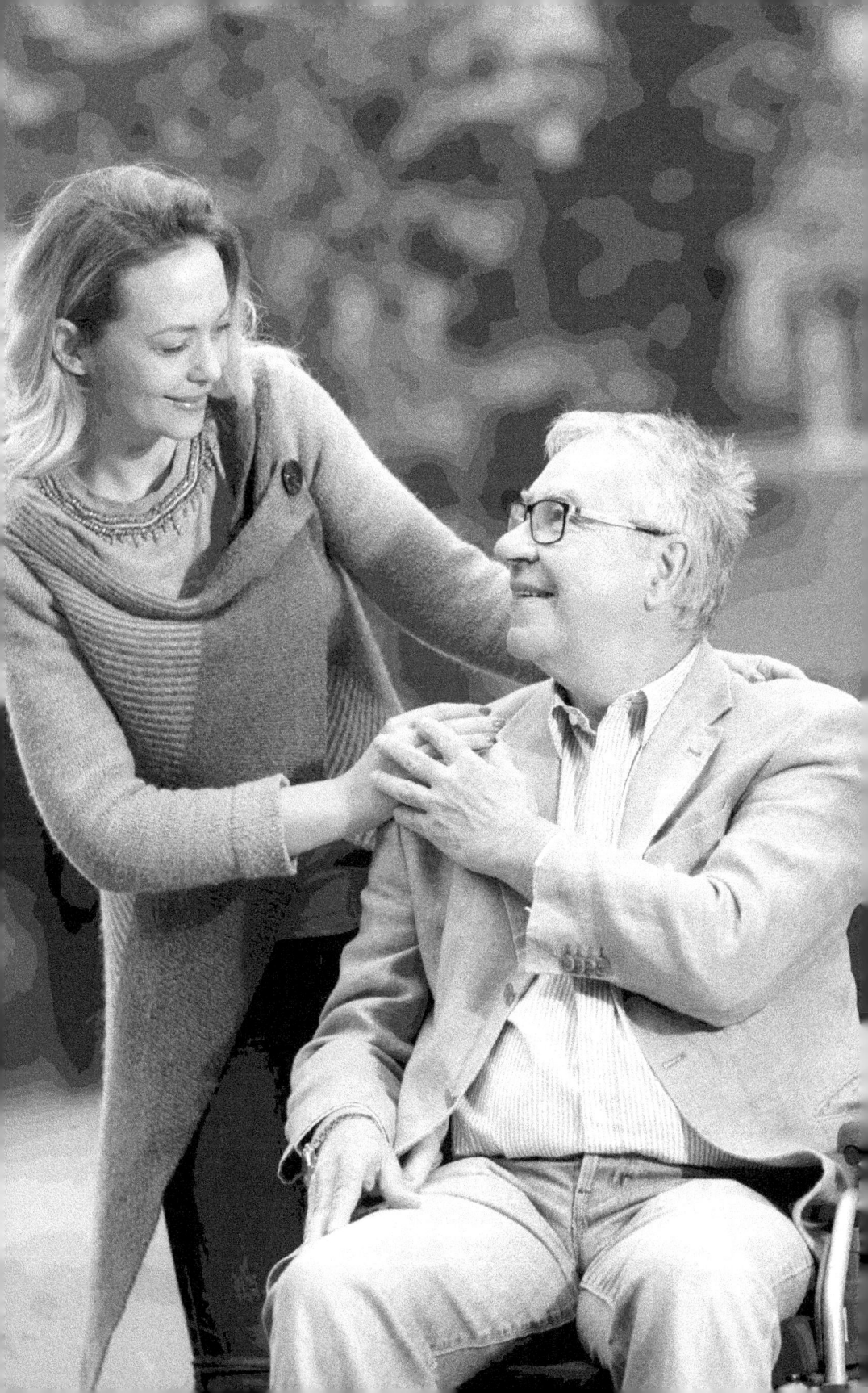

Chapter Ten.
Empowerment Through Knowledge

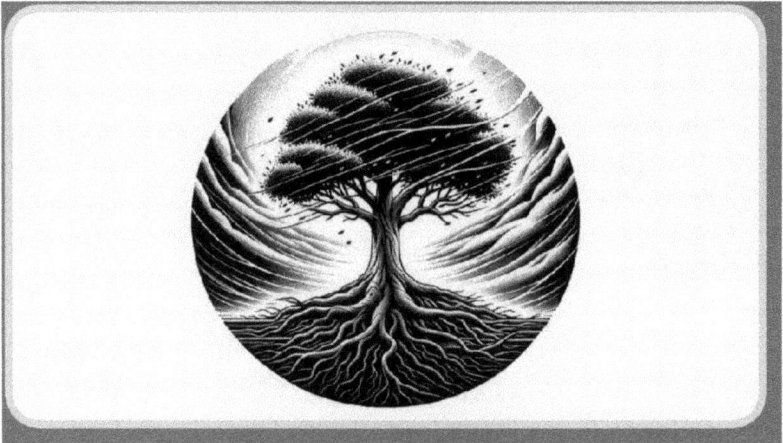

"A hero is an ordinary individual who finds the strength to persevere and endure despite overwhelming obstacles."

–Christopher Reeve.

Equipping Caregivers for Excellence

Imagine walking into a space where every corner holds a promise of growth and where every interaction is a step towards excellence. That is the essence of empowering caregivers. We are not just talking about giving them tools; we are talking about arming them with knowledge. Knowledge that not only enriches their ability to care but also elevates their confidence to new heights.

Now, let's dive deep into the world of caregiving. A caregiver's role is pivotal. It is demanding, both emotionally and physically. Yet, it remains one of the most rewarding jobs. Knowing how to perform this role beautifully is not just about instincts; it's about being equipped with the right knowledge. This is the groundwork for providing outstanding care. How, you ask? Let's unfold this together.

Firstly, think about a time when you stood before a challenge, uncertain about the next step. Now, think about how you felt after learning exactly what to do. That sense of relief, power, and readiness is priceless, isn't it? That's exactly what knowledge does for caregivers. It transforms them from being uncertain helpers to becoming competent and assured providers of care.

Education in caregiving does more than just teach. It changes the very fabric of caregiving quality. Consider a caregiver who understands the nuances of patient communication, recognizes the subtleties of non-verbal cues, and adapts seamlessly to the changing needs of their patient. This level of intuition comes from a sound education that is ongoing and responsive to the demands of the caregiving field.

Continuous learning is not a fancy term we throw around. It's a necessity. The world is always turning, and with it, the needs and best practices of caregiving also evolve. To stay ahead, to provide the best care, and to build a fortress of confidence around oneself, a caregiver must remain a student at heart. Why is this so important? Well, imagine the sense of accomplishment that comes from knowing you're doing the right thing, at the right time, for the right reasons. This is the confidence that education breeds in caregivers. It's the type of assurance that doesn't waver in the face of adversity. Caregivers who invest in their knowledge base are building a foundation that will support both them and their patients for years to come.

Let's consider the practical side of this empowerment. When caregivers engage in learning, whether through books, seminars, or hands-on training, they acquire a toolbox brimming with strategies and solutions for a myriad of situations. They become not just reactive, but proactive. They can anticipate issues and address them before they escalate. They are no longer just participants in the caregiving process; they become leaders in it.

We cannot overstate the benefits of continuous learning in the caregiving field. It is the golden thread that weaves through every aspect of excellent care. It is the difference between a good caregiver and an exceptional one. It is the armor that guards against burnout and the beacon that lights the path to personal and professional satisfaction.

To bring all these ideas together, let's put it straightforwardly: Equipping caregivers with knowledge is not optional, it is essential. It is the root from which grows the sturdy tree of excellence. Every piece of information, every skill learned, and every insight gained is a nutrient that feeds this tree, allowing it to flourish and provide the shade of confidence and care under which patients can thrive. It is through this detailed and thorough approach to knowledge that caregivers can stand tall, knowing they are providing the best care possible. They can look at themselves in the mirror and say with certainty, "I am equipped for excellence."

And while the journey to knowledge is a personal one, it is also a collective effort. By sharing their learning and experiences, caregivers contribute to a community of practice that uplifts the entire profession. In this way, the empowerment of one becomes the empowerment of many, and the cycle of excellence continues to revolve, lifting everyone it touches to new and greater heights.

As we move forward, let's keep in mind that this is just the beginning. The path of knowledge is infinite, and there is always more to learn, more to understand, and more to apply. This chapter is dedicated to the pursuit of that knowledge, and to the caregivers who seek it with a fervent and unwavering spirit.

Accessing and Utilizing Resources

Let's talk about something important. Really important. You see, when it comes to caring for someone, having the right information at your fingertips can be a game-changer. Now, I want to tell you about the many ways you can find helpful information and support. This is big. This will help you become the best caregiver you can be.

First off, there are books. Ah, books. They are like treasure chests of knowledge waiting to be opened. You can find books written by experts who've spent their lives understanding what you're going through. These books can give you tips, tell you stories, and teach you about caring for someone with special needs. When you read a book, take notes. Jot down what stands out to you. Keep those notes. They will come in handy, trust me.

Then, we have online courses. The internet is full of them. Online courses can guide you step by step. They show you how to do things right. You can watch videos, do exercises, and even talk to others who are learning just like you. It's like being in a class, but you're at home in your comfy pants. And you can go back and watch parts again if you need to. Isn't that neat?

Support groups are next on our list. These are groups of people who are all caring for someone. They meet up, they talk, and they help each other. They share what they know, and they listen. Finding a support group can be as easy as looking online or asking your doctor. Being in a group like this means you're not alone. Others are there. They get it.

What about professional associations? Yes, they are a thing too. Professional associations are like clubs for people who work in care. They have resources, training, and people you can talk to. They keep up with all the new stuff in the world of caregiving. Joining one can make you feel like a pro because you're surrounded by pros. It's a smart move.

Now, let's get down to how you really use all these resources. It's not just about having them. It's about making them work for you. So, when you get a new book, don't just put it on the shelf. Open it. Read a chapter a day. Make it a part of your routine, like your morning coffee.

With online courses, find the ones that fit your schedule. Do a little each day. Set goals, like finishing one section a week. Stick to it. And if there's a forum or a place to chat with other students, get in there. Ask questions. Answer questions. Be a part of the community.

In support groups, be active. Go to meetings. Talk. Listen. These are your people. They know what you're going through. You can learn a lot from them, and they can learn from you too. Give support and take support. It's a beautiful thing.

Professional associations often have events and conferences. These are gold mines of information. Go to them whenever you can. Take notes. Lots of notes. Meet people. Build a network. These connections can be lifelines when you need advice or help down the road.

Here's the bottom line: caregiving is a big job. It's a challenging job. But you've got this. Because now you know about all these resources. And you know how to use them. This isn't just about finding information; it's about using it to do something amazing—to care in the best way you can, to make a difference in someone's life. That's what this is all about. So, what's your next step? Pick a resource. Any resource. Dive in. Learn. Grow. And remember, you're not just doing this for the person you're caring for; you're doing it for yourself, too. Because you deserve to feel confident and supported in what you do. And that, my friend, is just the beginning. Welcome to a world where you're empowered by knowledge, and where you have the tools to be the very best caregiver. It starts today, right here, with what you've just learned. Go and use it. Make it count.

And hey, while you're at it, why not join our community? We have newsletters, online courses, and all sorts of goodies for caregivers like you. Becoming a member means you're not just staying on top of your game; you're also part of a family. A family that looks out for each other, shares tips, and cheers each other on. We're all on this journey together.

Imagine finishing your day knowing you've got a whole team backing you up. That's the power of our community, and we're just a click away. We are ready to welcome you with open arms. So subscribe, follow, and let's embark on this journey of empowerment together. Remember, caring for someone is a big job, but with the right resources and a community like ours, you can do it—and you can do it well.

Finally, take a look at our 9-Step Calm Caregiving Course. It's packed with valuable insights just for you. And if you like bundles, we've got those too: workbooks, nurturing articles, audio, slides, videos, and so much more. All of this provides resources and information to make your caregiving journey smoother and more effective. It's about giving you quality value that sparks your interest and keeps you coming back for more.

SCAN THIS AND BOOK A FREE DISCOVERY
CALL NOW

So there you go. You've got a whole world of resources at your fingertips. Use them. Learn from them. Share them. And grow. You're a caregiver, and that's a special thing. With these tools, you'll not only survive but thrive. And that's a beautiful thing.

Advocating for Patients and Self

When you care for someone with dementia, you become their voice. They may struggle to tell doctors what they feel or need. It's up to you, the caregiver, to speak up. To tell doctors, nurses, and others what your patient needs. This is called advocating. It's a big word for helping someone get what they need.

But advocating isn't just about talking; it's also about listening. You need to listen to what your patient says, even when their words are hard to understand. You also need to listen to what doctors and nurses say, so you can ask the right questions. This helps you learn what your patient needs for their health.

Advocating is not always easy. Sometimes doctors are busy. They may not listen the first time. You may need to repeat what you say. You may need to be firm. It's like being a gentle bulldozer. You push, but you do it with a smile. This helps your patient get the best care.

Being a caregiver also means you need to take care of yourself. If you're tired or sick, you can't help someone else. So, you need to ask for help when you need it. Maybe a friend can sit with your patient while you rest, or maybe you can join a support group. This is also advocating. It's advocating for you.

Advocating can make you feel strong. It can give you the power to make sure your patient and you are treated well. When you know you can speak up and get help, it can make you feel good. It can make you feel like you can do anything. And that is very important.

So remember, advocating means speaking and listening. It means being kind while also being firm. It means caring for your patient and for yourself. And it's a big part of being a good caregiver.

Now, let's talk about how to do this well. There are some steps you can take to be a good advocate. First, you need to know what your patient wants and needs. This means talking to them, watching them, and understanding them. Once you know what they need, you can start to speak up for them.

When you talk to doctors or nurses, be clear. Speak in a strong voice. Look them in the eye. Tell them exactly what your patient needs. If they don't listen, tell them again. Don't give up. Keep going until they hear you.

It's also helpful to write things down. You can make a list of questions before you see the doctor. You can write down what the doctor says. This helps you remember. It also shows the doctor that you're serious about getting the best care for your patient.

There's one more thing to remember: you're not alone. There are many caregivers like you. You can talk to them. You can share stories and advice. You can help each other. This can make you feel strong. It can make you feel like part of a team. And that can help you advocate even better.

In the end, advocating is about love. It's about caring so much for someone that you will do whatever it takes to help them. It's about being strong for someone else. And that is a beautiful thing.

So, keep speaking up. Keep listening. Keep caring for your patient and for yourself. This is the heart of being a caregiver. And it's what makes you so important. Advocating for patients and yourself is a path to well-being for everyone involved. It's not just a duty; it's a privilege. And it's an essential part of the journey you're on as a caregiver. By following these steps, you ensure that both your patient and you have a voice in the caregiving process, leading to better outcomes and a stronger sense of empowerment. So, use your voice, write down your thoughts, join hands with others, and never forget the power of advocacy in the caregiving journey.

Staying Informed and Up-to-Date

Imagine you're walking through a garden. You look around and see flowers blooming, and bees buzzing, and you feel the warmth of the sun on your skin. Just like a garden, the world of dementia care is always growing and changing. New ideas pop up like flowers. They can make the care we give better and the lives of those with dementia brighter. But to see these changes, just like the flowers, we need to keep our eyes open.

Knowledge is like water for the garden. It helps everything grow. For caregivers, fresh knowledge keeps skills sharp and minds clear. It's important to drink in new information. How do we do that? We can read newsletters, join groups, and go to workshops. These are our gardening tools in the world of caregiving.

First, let's talk about newsletters. They're like letters from a friend who always has something new to share. When you subscribe to a good newsletter about dementia care, it's like getting a regular update on what's new and helpful. It can tell you about new ways to make meals easier for someone with dementia or how to keep their minds active and happy. This is important because what we knew yesterday may not be the best thing for today. And what works today might be even better tomorrow. Newsletters keep us close to the heartbeat of new discoveries and ideas.

Imagine you have a question about dementia care. Where do you go? You could join a professional network. Think of it as a big family of caregivers. Everyone shares what they know. They talk about what works and what doesn't. In this family, you can ask your questions and get answers from people who have been in your shoes. They understand the ups and downs of caregiving. By sharing stories and advice, everyone gets stronger and smarter. It's like each person in the network is a gardener, and together, they help the whole garden thrive.

Workshops are another great way to learn. They're like classes where you can see, touch, and practice new things. Let's say there's a workshop on how to help someone with dementia sleep better. In the workshop, you might learn about calming music or a new kind of night light. You get to ask questions and try things out. Sometimes, you even get to meet the people who come up with these new ideas. Workshops can be a fun day out, and you come home with new tools to make caregiving a little bit easier.

Why is staying informed so important? Because the world doesn't stand still, and neither does dementia. Researchers are always working to understand it better. They study the brain, they try new medicines, and they look for ways to make life smoother for those with dementia and their caregivers. When we stay informed, we bring the best of these new ideas into our daily care. It's like we're always adding new tools to our toolkit. This means better care for the people we love and less guessing for us. It's a win-win.

So, how do we stay informed? It's as simple as signing up for a newsletter, joining a network, or going to a workshop. This might sound like a lot, but think about it like watering a garden. You don't do it all at once. You water a little bit each day. So, take a small step today. Sign up for one newsletter. Tomorrow, maybe check out a professional network. The day after, look for a workshop to attend. Little by little, you'll find your caregiving garden flourishing with new life and possibilities.

Remember, when we learn about new ideas in dementia care, we're not just filling our heads with facts. We're growing as caregivers. We're making life better for the people we care for. We're turning care into a beautiful garden that blooms with love, understanding, and the very best of what we know. So, let's grab our gardening tools—our newsletters, networks, and workshops—and get ready to grow.

As you take these steps, you're not just staying on top of what's new. You're becoming a beacon of hope and help. You show others that caring for someone with dementia is important and that they are always getting better. As you grow in your caregiving journey, remember that each piece of new information is a seed of change. Plant it in your care and watch as it grows into something beautiful—a better life for both you and those you care for. That's the power of staying informed and up-to-date. That's the power of knowledge in dementia care.

Building Confidence Through Learning

Education is a shining beacon in the journey of caregiving. It lights the path and guides the caregiver through the twists and turns of their noble vocation. Learning is not just about accumulating facts; it's a transformative process that builds confidence. This confidence is not the loud and boastful kind. It's a quiet certainty that comes from knowledge.

Let's think about what it means to learn. To learn is to understand new things in a way that makes you feel sure and strong. When caregivers learn, they find out how to do their job better. They find out how to take care of someone who needs them. This is important work. It's work that can change lives.

But where does one start? The world is full of places to learn. There are books, and there are classes. There are videos, and there are websites. Each one is a treasure chest waiting to be opened. Inside, there are answers to questions and solutions to problems. Caregivers can reach out and take this treasure. They can make it their own.

When a caregiver learns something new, it's like getting a key. This key can unlock doors. Behind these doors, there are better ways to care for those who depend on them. There is understanding, and there is comfort. There is also a new kind of power—the power to do good in the best way possible. This is the power of knowing.

Knowledge brings skill, and skill brings confidence. A caregiver who learns becomes more sure of themselves. They know what to do when a new challenge comes. They can stand tall and face it, not because they are not afraid, but because they are prepared. They have learned, and because they have learned, they are strong.

It's not always easy to find the time to learn. Lives are busy, and days are short. But even a little learning can make a big difference. A few minutes spent reading a helpful article can reveal a better way to help someone stand or walk. A short conversation with another caregiver can share a secret to calming a worried heart. These are small steps, but they lead to big places. Every chance to learn is precious. It's like finding a piece of a puzzle.

Caregivers can look for these pieces. They can fit them together. Slowly, a picture starts to form. It's a picture of how to give care that is kind and smart. This picture can guide them as they work each day.

Educational opportunities are all around. They call out to caregivers to come and learn. There are formal classes that lead to certificates and degrees. These are shiny badges of honor that say, "I know." There are also informal talks and groups where caregivers share their stories and their wisdom. Here, a listening ear can learn much.

One might wonder why learning is so tied to confidence. The answer is simple. When caregivers learn, they understand not just the "what" but the "why." They see the reasons behind the actions they take. This deep understanding is the root of true confidence. It's the difference between following a recipe and being a chef. The chef knows the flavors and the science. The chef can create and adapt because they have knowledge. This is the goal of learning in caregiving—to become the chef, not just the cook.

Learning is a journey with no end. The world changes and grows, and so must the caregiver. New discoveries are made. New methods are taught. Caregivers can keep up if they keep learning. They can be ready for the future and all it brings. The key is to never stop looking for knowledge. Never stop growing. Never stop becoming more than you were the day before.

In the end, it's not just about the caregiver. It's about the ones they care for. It's about giving them a life that is full and happy. It's about being the best caregiver one can be. A caregiver armed with knowledge and brimming with confidence is a powerful force. They can make a world of difference in the lives of those they touch.

So, to the caregivers out there, I say this: reach out for learning. Grab it with both hands. Take it into your heart. Let it fill you with confidence. Then go out and use what you've learned to make the world a better place. One act of caring at a time.

Recap: Knowledge is Power

By now, we've taken a thorough stroll through the maze of caregiving, haven't we? We've looked at each twist and turn, uncovering the tools and tricks that make for an effective caregiver. It's been quite the journey, full of insights and learning. But this is not just any journey. It's one that strengthens you with every step you take. Let's pause for a moment and think about that strength. It comes from knowledge. Knowledge you've gained by reading, listening, and practicing. And with this power, you're not just taking care of someone else; you're also taking care of yourself.

Let's revisit what we've learned, but not in a hurried manner. No, we'll take it slow, ensuring you grasp each vital piece. In these moments, remember that it's not just about recalling information. It's about understanding why this knowledge is crucial and how it can transform your caregiving experience.

Think of it as a map. With this map, you're not wandering aimlessly; you're navigating with purpose and confidence. You've learned that equipping yourself with knowledge is like having a key. It unlocks the best care you can provide. And not just that, it opens doors to confidence that might have seemed shut tight before. Remember how you felt when you first began this chapter? Now think about how you feel, knowing what you know. There's a difference, right? That difference is empowerment.

Now, to keep that feeling strong, you must use your resources. Think about those books you've stacked up, the online courses you've bookmarked, and the support groups you've noted down. These aren't just names on a list. They're your allies in caregiving. When you use these resources, you're not just learning; you're enhancing your ability to provide the best care possible.

Advocating for your patients and yourself is not a simple task. But now, with the skills you've developed, it's not daunting either. You've learned techniques to speak up effectively. Every time you communicate your needs or the needs of those you care for, you're building a bridge to better care. That's something to be proud of. Self-advocacy is not just about speaking out; it's about ensuring your voice is heard, respected, and acted upon.

Staying informed is like keeping the tools in your belt sharp and ready. You've learned the importance of keeping up with the latest in dementia care. It's not just about reading the latest news or attending workshops. It's about ensuring that your care is always at the cutting edge, and that you're ready for whatever comes your way. This isn't just about staying informed; it's about staying ahead.

And then, there's the role of confidence in your learning journey. It's the thread that ties everything together. With each new piece of knowledge, your confidence grows. This isn't just theoretical. It's real. It's the feeling you have when faced with a challenge and knowing, deep down, that you have the tools to meet it head-on. That's the true power of learning.

Moving Forward: Your Action Plan

So, what can you do to keep this momentum going? Here's a checklist, a sort of action plan, if you will. These steps are your next moves to maintain the empowerment you now hold:

- **Review your notes** from this chapter regularly. This keeps the information fresh and at the forefront of your mind.

- **Set aside time each week** to read or watch something related to caregiving. It could be an article, a chapter from a book, or a video tutorial.

- **Join a new online course or webinar** on caregiving every few months. This introduces you to new concepts and skills.

- **Connect with other caregivers**, either in person or online. Sharing experiences reinforces your own knowledge and provides emotional support.

- **Keep a journal** of your caregiving experiences. Reflect on what you learn from each situation. This is personal research that's invaluable.

- **Subscribe to a caregiving newsletter or magazine**. This ensures that the latest developments come straight to you.

- **Attend a workshop or conference** at least once a year. These are great opportunities to learn from experts and peers alike.

- **Advocate for your care recipient and yourself** when necessary. Use the techniques you've learned to be an effective voice.

- **Teach others**. Sharing your knowledge not only helps others but also reinforces what you've learned.

As you move forward, remember that knowledge isn't static. It grows, it evolves, and as it does, so do you. Each piece of information you absorb, every skill you develop, turns you not just into a better caregiver but into a stronger individual as well.

Never forget that this power you hold, the power of knowledge, doesn't wane. It only gets stronger with use. So use it, nurture it, and watch as it transforms not only your life but the lives of those around you. It's more than just caregiving. It's about creating a world of care that's informed, compassionate, and unyielding. It's about standing strong in a role that many depend on, but few truly understand its depth.

You, my friend, are now among those few. Take this knowledge, wield it wisely, and go forth with the assurance that you are providing the best care possible. Because when you know better, you do better. And isn't that what we're all striving for?

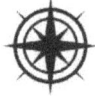

Chapter Eleven
Defining Hope in Dementia Care.

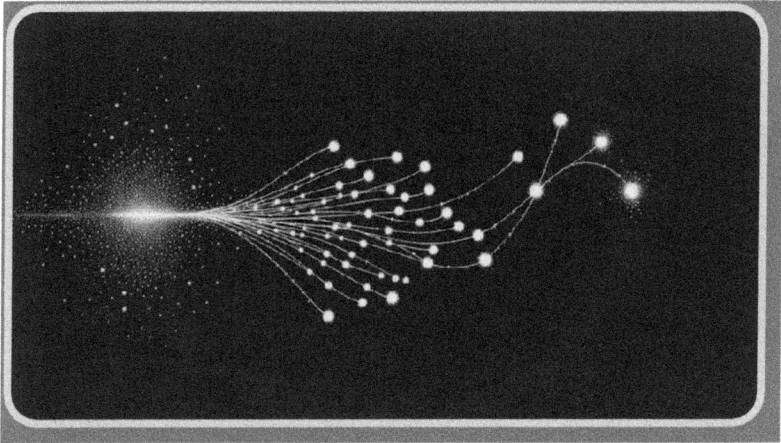

"We can all make a difference in the lives of others in need because it is the simplest of gestures that make the most significant of differences."

– Miya Yamanouchi

Defining Hope in Dementia Care

You know hope is a Big Deal. Especially when we talk about taking care of people with dementia. It's like having a light in a dark room. It helps care partners and those with dementia find the strength to keep going. So, let's talk about what hope means in this special setting. In dementia care, hope is holding onto the belief that good things can happen, even when times are tough. It's seeing the person beyond their illness. It's about staying positive and looking for the bright spots on difficult days.

Why is hope so important for caregivers? Well, it keeps them going. It helps them wake up every day, ready to help and make a difference. Without hope, the hard work of caregiving can feel too heavy. But with hope, everything seems a bit lighter. And for those with dementia, hope can mean feeling safe, cared for, and valued, no matter how much the disease affects them.

The Impact of Hope on Well-being

Now, let's take a slow walk through the garden of well-being and see how hope helps it bloom. When caregivers and those with dementia have hope, they can handle stress better. They can enjoy moments more. They can smile, laugh, and feel close to each other, even when times are tough.

For those with dementia, having a hopeful caregiver can make all the difference. It can mean feeling calm instead of scared. It can mean feeling happy instead of sad. And for caregivers, hope can help them stay healthy. With hope, they can sleep better, eat better, and take better care of themselves. This means they can keep being there for the person they care for. It means they can keep making each day as good as it can be for both of them.

In short, hope is powerful. It's like a special medicine for the heart and mind. It helps both caregivers and those with dementia to live better lives. It's something we can all give and get, and it doesn't cost a thing. By understanding hope, we can all help make each other's lives a bit brighter, a little at a time.

So, to wrap up, hope is more than just a word. It's a force, a vital tool, that can shape the journey through dementia care. It's something to hold onto, share, and nurture every day. And that's what we'll keep talking about: how to keep that hope alive and make it grow for you and the person you care for. Because when there's hope, there's a way to keep moving forward together.

Cultivating Hope in Everyday Care

Hope. It's a small word, but it holds a big place in our lives, especially when caring for someone with dementia. Hope is like a light in a dark room. It can make a big difference. When you're caring for someone with dementia, finding hope might seem hard at times. But it's there, in the everyday moments, waiting to be found and held onto.

Let's talk about small wins and celebrations first. A small win can be as simple as a smile, a word, or even a moment of calm. It's important to notice these things. They matter. When you're taking care of someone each day, these are the moments that can give you strength. And celebrating them helps. You could keep a journal or just take a moment at the end of the day to think about the good parts. This helps you remember that even on tough days, there are still good moments.

How do we make these moments of hope a part of our daily lives? It's simple: we look for them, and we remember to celebrate them. If the person you're caring for has a good morning, that's a win. Maybe they remembered something, or they laughed at an old joke. That's something to be happy about. When you notice these small wins, say it out loud or write it down. Share it with friends or family. This helps make the win feel real, and it spreads hope to others, too.

But why does celebrating these small wins matter? Well, it's like watering a plant. If you water a plant, it grows. If you notice and celebrate the good moments, your hope grows, too. And when hope grows, it makes it easier to get through the hard days. Remember, even the smallest win is still a win. It's like finding a penny on the ground. It might not be much, but it's still something good.

Moving on to future-focused care planning, this is about making plans that give you and the person with dementia something to look forward to. It's like marking a calendar with a fun event in the future, but for care. These plans don't have to be big. They can be small, like enjoying a favorite meal next week or visiting a friend. The point is to have something on the horizon that brings a spark of joy.

How do we do this? You start by thinking of what the person you're taking care of enjoys. Then, you make a plan to include that in the future. It could be as simple as a special snack on Friday or a phone call with a loved one on Sunday. It's about having little things to look forward to together. It's a way of saying, "Yes, there's something good coming up. Let's get ready for it." This helps both of you keep moving forward, looking ahead instead of only seeing the troubles of today.

Why is this important? When we have something to look forward to, it's like a light at the end of a tunnel. It helps us keep going. It's not about ignoring the hard parts of dementia care; it's about balancing them with moments of light. Planning for the future, even in small ways, can be a powerful tool to bring hope into everyday care.

Remember, hope is something we all need, and it's something we can all create. By celebrating small wins and making future-focused plans, we bring hope into the everyday. We make each day a little brighter for ourselves and for those we care for with dementia. It's about finding joy in the journey, even when the path is hard. And when we do this, we're not just caring for someone. We're nurturing hope, and that, my friend, is a beautiful thing.

To sum it all up, keep your eyes open for those little moments of victory. They are like treasures hidden in your day. And make plans for good things to come. They are like stars in the night sky, guiding you forward. Hope is there in the everyday care you give. It's there for you to find, to hold onto, and to grow. And that's something truly special.

Communicating Hope

Hope is like a light. When you care for someone with dementia, you hold a torch that lights up the dark paths they might see ahead. It's not just about what you do or what you say; it's about how you make them feel.

Hopeful communication is a way of talking to someone that brings out this light and helps them feel safe and positive, even when things are tough.

To communicate hope, start by smiling. A smile is a simple act, but it is powerful. It can light up a room. It can warm a heart. When you smile at someone with dementia, you're not just using your lips and teeth. You're sending a message. You're saying, "I'm here with you. I believe in you. We can find happiness, even in small moments." And often, they will smile back. That's a moment of connection. It's a spark of hope.

Next, use words that are warm and kind. Choose words that can wrap around someone, like a cozy blanket. Instead of saying, "Don't be sad," you can say,

"I'm here with you. Let's find something that makes you happy." This is important. The words "don't be sad" focus on sadness. But when you talk about finding happiness, you point to something bright and good. You're guiding them towards hope without dismissing their feelings.

But it's not just about the words. It's about listening—really listening. When someone with dementia talks, give them your full attention. Look them in the eyes. Nod your head. Make little sounds that say, "I hear you. I understand." This shows respect. It shows you value what they have to say. It can make them feel like they still have a voice that matters. And that can help them hold on to hope.

Every day, you can find ways to help those with dementia feel hope. Encourage them to talk about the good times. Help them remember happy memories. You can say, "Tell me about a time when you felt really happy." When they share, listen with all your heart. Their stories are like treasures. They remind them of joy. They remind them that life is still full of good things. And when it's hard for them to remember, you can help. You can say, "I remember when you told me about your garden. You loved the roses." Sharing memories like this can light up their face. It's like you're holding their hand and walking them back to a sunny day full of beautiful flowers. You're helping them see that the beauty they once loved is still with them—in their memories and in your shared stories.

Another Way to Share Hope

Another way to share hope is by setting small goals. You can do this by saying, "Let's work on this puzzle together. I bet we can finish it by lunchtime." Goals like this are like little bridges. They help the person with dementia walk from feeling unsure to feeling like they can do something good. And when you reach the goal, it's a celebration. It's proof that they can still achieve things. And that can make hope grow.

It's also good to share news about friends and family. Talk about the good things happening to people they care about. Say, "Guess what? Your grandson scored a goal in his soccer game!"

This kind of news connects them to the world outside. It reminds them that life around them is still full of good news, and it makes them feel part of it. Feeling connected is like having roots. It helps hope stay strong, even when the wind blows hard.

And sometimes, hope is about the little things. It's about holding a hand. It's about sitting together in silence, looking at the sky. It's about playing their favorite song and watching their eyes light up. These moments are small, but they are like stars in the night sky. They might be tiny, but they shine brightly. They remind us that there is always something beautiful to be found, even in the dark.

Lastly, remember to take care of your own hope. When you are hopeful, it's easier to share that hope. Do things that fill you with joy and peace. Take breaks when you need them. Talk to friends. Laugh. Rest. When your heart is full of hope, you'll be like a lighthouse. Your hope will shine and show the way for others, especially for those with dementia who look to you for guidance and comfort.

So, keep hope alive in your words, in your actions, and in your heart. Communicate hope in every smile, every story, and every moment of understanding. Believe that this hope you nurture will make a real difference in the lives of those you care for. It's not just about facing today. It's about looking forward to tomorrow with a heart full of light and a spirit ready to find joy in the journey, no matter what it brings.

Hope-Building Strategies for Caregivers

When you spend your days caring for someone with dementia, you might find yourself getting tired. It's not just your body that feels it; it's your heart and mind too. It can be tough—really tough. But there is something powerful that can help, and it's as light as a feather and as strong as steel. That powerful thing is hope. Let's talk about how you, as a caregiver, can hold onto hope even when the days are long.

First, let's talk about personal resilience. It's like being a strong tree in a big storm. The wind blows hard, but the tree stands firm. You can be like that tree. Building resilience means that, when things get hard, you don't break. Instead, you bend and then you rise back up again. Here's a way to do that: take care of yourself.

Yes, you. You are just as important as the person you're caring for. Every day, find a little time for yourself. It could be a few minutes sitting outside, a short walk, or a cup of tea while you watch the sunrise. These moments are like deep breaths for your soul. They recharge you and give you the strength to face the day. And when you face the day strong, hope shines brighter. Always remember that you can't pour from an empty cup, so fill yours first.

Now, let's talk about optimism and realism. You see, being a caregiver means you know the truth about dementia. You know it's a tough road. That's being realistic. But being optimistic means you see the good in each day, no matter how small. It's like looking at the sky at night. Yes, it's dark, but oh, look at those stars! To balance realism and optimism, you focus on what you can do, not what you can't. You celebrate every good moment, every smile, and every word. You find joy in the little things, and that joy builds hope.

Building hope doesn't mean you ignore the hard stuff. No, it means you face it, but you don't let it take over. It's like having an umbrella in the rain. The rain is still there, but you stay dry. You protect your hope as that umbrella protects you. You acknowledge the rain, but you also know it will pass and that there will be sunny days again.

Let's also think about your words. The words you say to yourself are powerful. They're like seeds you plant in a garden. If you plant seeds of worry, you'll grow a garden of fears. But if you plant seeds of hope, you'll grow a garden of possibilities. Start with what you tell yourself in the morning. Say, "Today may have challenges, but I can handle them." Believe in your own strength. Believe in the difference you're making. Those beliefs, those words—they're the sunlight and water helping your hope grow.

Lastly, let's talk about community. You're not alone. There are so many others like you, caring and hoping. Reach out to them. Share your stories, your struggles, and your successes. When you share, you find out you're part of a big, caring family. And families stick together. They hold each other up. When you're feeling low, someone else's hope can lift you. When you're strong, your hope can lift someone else up. Together, you all become a forest of strong trees, standing tall through every storm.

In your days as a caregiver, remember these things: take care of yourself, find the balance between optimism and realism, watch your words, and lean on your community. Do these, and you'll build hope like a master craftsman builds a house—strong and sure. And in that house of hope, you'll find comfort and strength for all your days. Keep going, keep caring, and keep hoping. It's worth it. It really is.

Overcoming Hopelessness

So, you might be feeling down. Maybe you're a caregiver, and you've hit a point where hope seems like a stranger. Or you're looking after someone with dementia, and it feels like the light at the end of the tunnel just flickered out. I'm here to talk about that, to help you find that spark again. It's tough, we know, but let's walk through this together.

First, let's talk about those signs of despair. It's important to get to know them. Someone might start saying things are pointless. They might stop doing things they used to love. They may even pull away from friends. These are like red flags, waving at us, telling us something's not right.

What we do next is just as important. We need to step in, but gently. It's like seeing a friend with a flat tire. You wouldn't just walk away; you'd offer to help. Same thing here. We reach out. We say, "I'm here for you." We listen. Sometimes, that's all someone needs—someone to just be there.

But what if that's not enough? Well, that's where support systems come in. Think of it like a team. You're not alone. There are groups, professionals, and others who get what you're going through. They're ready to hold your hand and pull you back up.

So, we connect. We find these groups. Maybe it's a local support circle. Or an online community. Places where people say, "I've been there. Let's talk." They share tips, hugs, and sometimes, just a cup of coffee and an understanding nod. It's all about knowing you're part of something bigger. A group that cares.

Now, here's the thing about hope. It's not just a fluffy cloud. It's solid. It's the belief that tomorrow could be a bit brighter, that the next step isn't into the darkness, but into a bit of light. And that's powerful. It can lift you up, keep you going, and spread to those you care for.

So, how do we build that hope back? Simple steps. We start by setting small goals. Not climbing a mountain, but maybe just taking a short walk or having a good talk with the person you're caring for. It's about those little wins. They add up, you know?

Another thing is celebrating. When anything good happens, no matter how tiny, we cheer. We say, "Hey, we did that!" It's like giving yourself a gold star. It feels good. And it reminds us that not everything is lost. There's still good stuff happening.

And let's not forget the power of just being present. Sometimes, the best thing we can do is just sit with someone. No words. Just being there, side by side. It's a silent way of saying, "You're not in this alone."

So, what's the takeaway? It's that hopelessness doesn't have to be the end of the story. It can be a tough chapter, sure. But it's not the last one. With the right moves, and the right support, you can turn the page. You can find that hope again, bit by bit. And you can share it with those who need it most.

It's okay to reach out for help. It's okay to say, "I'm struggling." There's strength in that. It's the first step toward climbing out of the pit of despair. And once you're out, you can help others, too. You can be the hand that pulls someone else into the light.

At the end of the day, it's about not giving up. It's about finding those little moments of joy and holding on to them. It's about knowing that, even when the sky is gray, the sun hasn't disappeared—it's just hiding behind the clouds. And it will shine again. You'll see.

So, let's wrap this up with a clear, actionable step. Today, find one small thing that gives you hope. Maybe it's a picture, a song, a memory. Hold onto it. Let it be your anchor. And then, reach out. Find a support group. Talk to a friend. Share your hope. And let their hope lift you, too.

Remember, you're not alone. There are resources, people, and tools waiting to help you. And together, we can nurture that spark of hope until it's a blazing fire, warming everyone around us. That's the journey we're on. And it's a journey worth taking.

And if you've found even a little bit of comfort or inspiration in what I've shared, consider joining our community. We've got newsletters, courses, and lots of support that can make this tough road a little easier. We're here for you, every step of the way.

Chapter Recap

Hope. We've talked a lot about it, haven't we? It's like a light that keeps shining, even when the room gets dark. In the world of dementia care, hope is what keeps us going. It helps us to wake up in the morning and say, "Today, I will make a difference." We've explored what hope means in this journey and learned that it's more than just a feeling. It's a tool, a resource, and a friend that walks with us, hand in hand, as we care for those who once cared for us.

Throughout this chapter, we looked at hope from every angle. We painted a picture of it not with colors, but with words. Words that showed us how hope can improve the lives of both caregivers and dementia patients. But it wasn't just about seeing hope; it was about feeling it, touching it, and making it part of our daily lives.

So, let's breathe in deeply. Let's take a moment to wrap up all that we've covered. We started by defining hope in the context of dementia care. We saw that hope is not a one-size-fits-all; it's personal and unique to each caregiver and patient. It's believing that good things can happen, despite the tough times.

The impact of hope on well-being is huge. It's like a domino effect; when hope is high, spirits are lifted, and this positivity can actually lead to better health outcomes. We've seen that hope is not just pie-in-the-sky thinking. It's powerful. It's real. And it works.

We then talked about how to plant seeds of hope in the everyday tasks of caring for someone with dementia. Recognizing and celebrating the small victories are like watering those seeds. It might be as simple as a smile from a loved one or a moment of clarity in their eyes. These are the wins that matter. Planning for the future with hope looks like setting goals—but not just any goals, achievable ones. Ones that give both caregivers and patients something to look forward to. It's about looking forward, even if it's just to the next meal, the next visit from a friend, or the next sunny day.

Communicating hope is like giving a gift every day. We do it with our words, our smiles, and our actions. We learned how to convey a sense of hope through our daily interactions and how to help patients catch that hope and hold onto it tightly.

Building personal resilience was a big topic too. It's about caregivers creating a well of hope inside themselves that they can draw from when times get tough. We need to balance being realistic with staying optimistic, which is like walking a tightrope with a safety net of hope stretched out below us.

Fighting off feelings of hopelessness is part of the journey, too. When hope starts to slip away, it's time to reach out to the support systems around us. The caregiver community is a treasure chest of hope. When we share our stories, we help to refill each other's cups of hope to the brim.

- **Now, let's make sure we remember all of this.** I have a checklist for you. It's a simple, follow-along guide to help you keep hope alive in your caregiving journey. Here are the steps:

- **Start each day by reminding yourself of one small thing you hope to see.** Maybe a moment of recognition, or a peaceful mealtime.

- **When you achieve a small win, take a moment to celebrate.** Share it with a friend, write it down, or just give yourself a mental high-five.

- **Set a small, achievable goal for the week.** Something to look forward to, like a walk in the park or a favorite meal for your loved one.

- **Choose your words with care, infusing hope into your conversations with everyone, especially your patient.**

- **Build your resilience.** Take care of yourself, so you can be a strong source of hope for others. This might mean taking a short break, reading a book, or enjoying a hobby.

- **If you feel your hope waning, don't be afraid to ask for help.** Call a friend, join a support group, or talk to a professional.

Finally, end each day by reflecting on what went well. Write down at least one thing that gave you hope. Collect these notes and look back on them when you need a boost.

Hope in dementia care is like a silent promise. It's a promise that we make to ourselves and to those we care for. It's the promise that, no matter what, we will not give up. We will fight for every good day, every peaceful moment, and every memory we can cherish. You've come a long way in understanding the role of hope in caregiving. Now, you can use this knowledge as a lantern to light the path ahead. And remember, you're not walking this path alone. We're right here with you, every step of the way.

Thank you for taking the time to read, learn, and grow. Your commitment to caring is a beacon of hope in itself. Keep shining, dear friend, and let that hope guide you through each day of your caregiving journey.

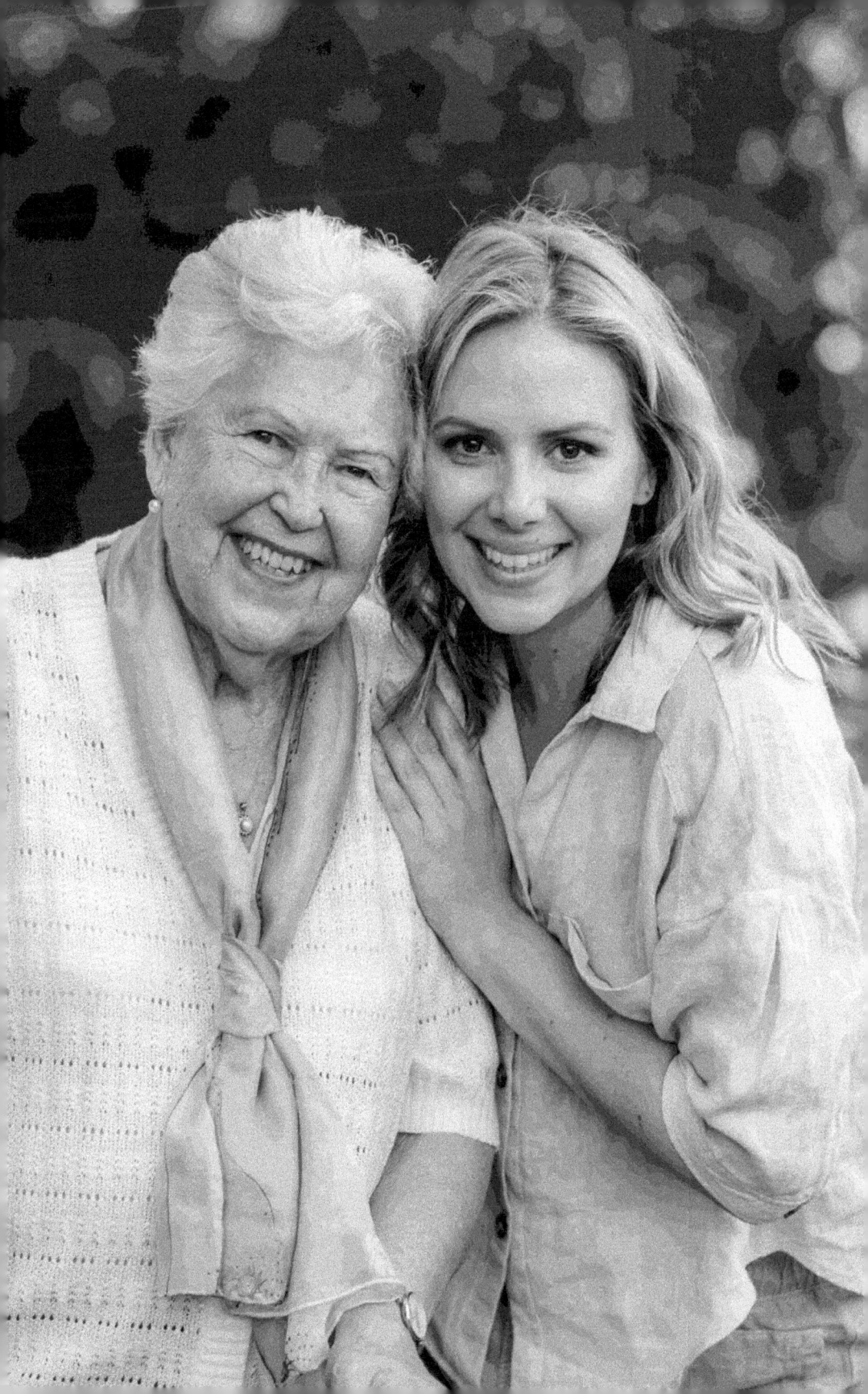

Conclusion.
Empowerment Through Knowledge

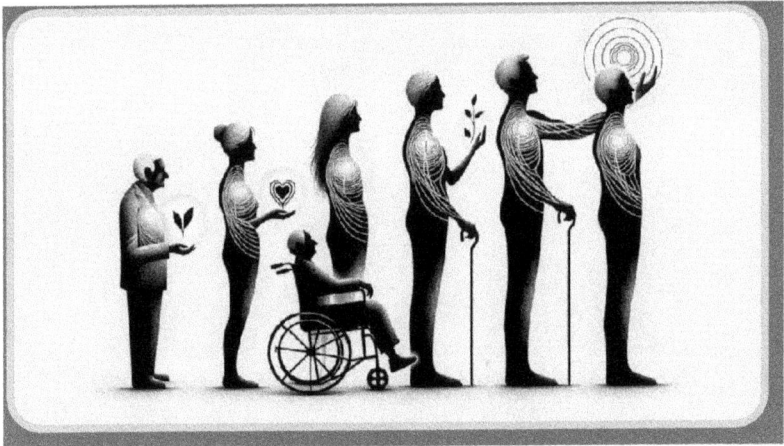

"There are only four kinds of people in the world. Those who have been caregivers. Those who are currently caregivers. Those who will be caregivers, and those who will need a caregiver."

– Rosalyn Carter

Equipping Caregivers for Excellence

Knowledge is a powerful tool. It is like a bright light in a dark room. It helps us see where we're going and what we need to do. For caregivers, knowledge is especially important.

Caregivers do a very special job. They help people who need extra care to live better lives. This could be someone who is very old, someone who is sick, or someone who cannot do some things by themselves. Caregivers need to know a lot to do their job well.

Let's talk about why knowing things is so important for caregivers. When you have the right information, you can make good choices. For example, if you are taking care of someone with a special kind of sickness, like dementia, you need to know about that sickness. You need to know what helps and what does not help. You need to know how to keep the person safe and happy. This is a big job, and it can be hard sometimes.

But here's the good news. When caregivers learn more, they can do their jobs better. They feel sure of themselves. They feel strong. They can help the person they are taking care of in the best way possible. But learning is not just about reading books or going to school. There are many ways to learn. You can talk to other caregivers. You can ask doctors and nurses questions. You can go to meetings or groups where people talk about caring for others. You can also look on the internet for really good places to learn more.

Knowing things helps caregivers in many ways. First, it helps them to understand the person they are taking care of. Every person is special. Every person has their own story. Caregivers need to know this story to help in the best way. They need to what makes the person happy or sad. They need to know what the person likes to do. All this information makes it easier to care for the person. It also makes the job more fun.

Another way knowledge helps is by making hard things easier. Sometimes, caregivers have to do things that are not easy. They might have to help the person get dressed or take a bath. They might have to give the person medicine. Or they might have to help the person remember things. When caregivers know the best ways to do these things, it is better for them and the person they are taking care of.

One more thing that is really important is safety. Caregivers need to keep the person they are taking care of safe. They also need to keep themselves safe. When caregivers know about safety, they can stop accidents before they happen. They can make the home a safe place. They can help the person move around without getting hurt. This is a very big part of the job.

So, you see, knowledge is like a toolbox. It is full of tools that can help caregivers do their job. It is full of ideas and ways to make things better. The more tools you have, the better you can do your job. And the better you can do your job, the happier you will be. And when you are happy, the person you are taking care of will be happy too. It is like a circle of happiness.

Now, let's talk about how to get this knowledge. It's not hard. You just have to look for it. You have to ask questions. You have to be curious. Think about what you want to know. Maybe you want to know how to make the person laugh. Maybe you want to know how to help them sleep better. Write down your questions. Then, look for the answers. You can find answers in many places. You can find them in books, online, or by talking to people who know a lot.

Remember, learning is a journey. It does not happen all at once. It takes time. Every day, you can learn something new. Every day, you can get better at your job. And as you learn, you will find that you feel more sure of yourself. You will feel like a superhero without a cape. You will be ready to help in the best way you can. And that is a wonderful thing.

So, let's make a plan. Let's decide to learn something new every day. Let's use the knowledge we get to do our job better. Let's share what we learn with other caregivers. Together, we can all do a great job. Together, we can all help the people we care for to live better lives. And together, we can all feel good about the work we do.

It's time to take the first step. It's time to start learning now. Let's open the door to knowledge and walk through it. On the other side, there is a world of good things waiting for us.

Accessing and Utilizing Resources

Think of a time when you needed help with something. Maybe it was a broken faucet at home or a flat tire on your car. You sought out the right tools and advice to fix the problem, right? Now, think about caregiving. Just like fixing that faucet or tire, caregivers need the right tools and good advice too. This is all about finding and using resources that can help.

First, let's talk about what resources are. Resources are things that give us help or support. They are like a friend who is always there to give us advice or a helpful book that has answers to our questions. For caregivers, these resources can be websites, books, local support groups, and even apps on your phone. They are full of useful information that can make caregiving a bit easier.

But where do you find these resources? One good place to begin is the internet. It can be a big help in finding things. You can look for websites that talk about taking care of people with dementia. These sites often have tips and stories from other caregivers. They can teach you new ways to help the person you are caring for. It's like finding a guidebook for the journey you're on.

Another place to find help is at the library. Libraries have lots of books. Some books are made just for caregivers. They can tell you how to do things, like make meals that are good for the person you're looking after. The people who work at the library can help you find these books. It's like going on a treasure hunt for helpful tips. Support groups are another kind of resource. These groups are for people who are doing the same thing as you—taking care of someone else. In these groups, people talk about their own stories. They share what works for them and what doesn't. It's like having a team of friends who understand what you're going through. You can find these groups by asking your doctor or looking online.

Apps on your phone can be resources too. Some apps remind you when to give medicine. Others help you keep track of doctor's appointments. There are even apps that can make you feel less alone by connecting you with other caregivers. These apps are like little helpers that you carry in your pocket. Now, why are these resources so important? Because they give you knowledge. And knowledge is like a power that can make you feel strong. When you know more, you can do things better. You can find new ways to solve problems. You can understand how to make the person you're caring for feel more comfortable. It's like learning how to score a point in a game—it helps you win.

Using these resources can also give you hope. Sometimes, caregiving can make you feel sad or tired. Reading a story from another caregiver can make you feel less alone. It can give you new energy to keep going. It's like the sun coming out after a lot of rainy days.

But it's not enough to just find these resources. You have to use them too. Think about it like a cookbook. If you just read a recipe but don't cook anything, you won't have a meal. You've got to use the recipe to make something. In the same way, you've got to use the tips and advice you find to make caregiving better.

Here's how you can start using these resources. Pick one day each week. Call it your 'Learning Day.' On this day, spend some time with one of the resources you found. Maybe you read a chapter from a caregiver's book. Or you could join a support group meeting. Or try a new app. Use this time to learn one new thing that can help you in caring.

Remember to take notes about what you learn. You can keep a small notebook or use your phone to write things down. This way, you won't forget the good ideas you find. It's like collecting coins that you can use later. After you learn something new, try it out. Maybe you read about a new way to keep the person you are caring for safe in their home. Give it a go. See if it works. And if it does, that's great! You've just made things better. If it doesn't work, that's okay too. You can try something else. It's all about trying and learning.

Lastly, talk about what you've learned with other people. You can share a good tip with another caregiver. Or tell your family about an app that helps you. By sharing, you help others too. It's like passing a ball in a game—it helps the whole team play better.

To wrap it up, finding and using resources can really help you as a caregiver. It can teach you new things, make you feel stronger, and give you hope. So start looking for these helpful tools today. Use them to make your caregiving journey a little easier. And remember, every little bit of knowledge you gain is like a step forward on this path. Keep walking and keep learning.

Advocating for Patients and Self

When we talk about taking care of others, especially those with conditions like dementia, there's something very important we need to remember. It's not just about giving medicines on time or making sure they're safe. It's about speaking up for them. That's called advocating. Advocating means asking for what someone needs and making sure they get it. It's like being a voice for someone who can't speak up loud enough on their own.

Now, let's think about why this is so important. People with dementia may sometimes not tell you what they need. They might be scared or not sure how to say it. That's where you come in. You know them well. You're with them a lot. You see things others don't. So you can help them a lot by telling doctors, nurses, and other people what the person you care for needs.

But it's not just about the person you're looking after. Advocating is for you too. When you take care of someone else, you must also take care of yourself. If you need help, it's okay to ask for it. If something doesn't feel right, say something. It's how you make sure you have the energy and health to keep on helping.

So, how do you do this? First, you learn. Learn about what dementia is, what it does, and how it changes things for people. There are books about it and websites too. Even doctors and nurses can teach you. When you know a lot, you can make better choices for the person with dementia.

Then, you talk. You talk to the people who can make things better. This could be doctors or people at places where your loved one goes, like a day care center. You tell them what's needed, like maybe a different medicine or a special kind of food. And you keep on talking until they listen. That's being a good advocate.

You also write things down. When did the medicine get given? How did they feel after? What did they eat? Writing it down helps you remember and it shows others what's going on. It's proof that can help you when you're advocating. Another part is being kind but strong. Some people might not listen at first.

They're busy or they don't understand. It doesn't mean you're wrong. Keep asking, keep explaining. Do it with kindness but be firm too. It's like knocking on a door until it opens. You don't bang it down, but you don't walk away either.

It's not just about talking. It's about listening too. Listen to what the person you're caring for is trying to tell you. It might not be with words. It could be the way they move or the looks on their faces. And listen to what the doctors and others tell you too. They know a lot. Together, you can all do more than any of you alone.

Sometimes, you might feel tired or like it's too much. That's okay. It happens to everyone. When that happens, find other people who understand. Maybe it's a group for caregivers or a friend who's been through the same thing. They can help you keep going.

Why is all this so important? Because when you advocate well, things get better. The person you're caring for gets what they need. They feel better and so do you.

You see, when you speak up, you're really saying, "I care. I want the best for you." And that's a powerful thing. It can change a lot, for them and for you.

Let's make it simple and clear. To be a good advocate, you learn, you talk, you write, you're kind but strong, and you listen. You do it for the person with dementia and you do it for yourself too. Because taking care means doing all these things. And when you do them well, you help a lot. You make lives better. And that's a very good thing to do.

Now, before we finish, let's not forget. If you're looking for more help or information, there's a lot out there. Books, websites, groups, and more. And if you're feeling like it's too much, reach out. There's always someone who can listen and help. That's part of taking care too. So, take a deep breath, get ready, and keep on advocating. It's worth it. You're worth it. And the person you care for is worth it too.

Staying Informed and Up-to-Date

Think about the world we live in today. Things change fast. New information pops up all the time. It's the same with caring for someone. To give the best care, we need to keep learning new things. This means staying up-to-date. This is super important when we take care of someone with dementia.

Now, let's talk about how to stay current with all the latest in dementia care. It's a bit like tending a garden. Just as a garden needs regular care to grow, your knowledge needs regular updates to thrive. It's not hard, really. But it does require you to take a few steps.

First, you should read often. There are articles, books, and websites full of information on dementia care. Reading helps you learn what's new and what works best. Look for trusted sources. These are places known for good, solid facts. They can be websites like www.Caregivers.today or www.Caregivers.coach.

Second, you can talk to experts. Experts are like your guides. They know a lot because they work with dementia every day. You can find them at talks, or you could even email them. Many love to share what they know. When you talk to experts, you learn a lot quickly.

Third, join groups with other caregivers. Other caregivers are like teammates. They understand what you're going through. They might know tips and tricks that you haven't heard about. Being in a group gives you support and information at the same time.

Fourth, attend workshops and seminars. These are special meetings where you learn hands-on. It's a bit like a class. You might practice new ways to help someone with dementia. Or learn about medicines and activities that are good for them.

Fifth, sign up for newsletters. Newsletters come to your email. They often have news about dementia care. They share stories from other caregivers. They might even tell you about events coming up that you can go to.

Doing these things keeps you sharp. It makes you a better caregiver. When you know what's new, you feel sure of yourself. You can do your job better. And when you do your job better, the person you care for feels better too.

But there's something else too. It's not just about learning. It's about using what you learn. When you learn a new fact, try it out. See if it works. If it does, great! If not, it's okay. You now know something that doesn't work. And that's also good to know.

So, to put it simply, staying informed and up-to-date is like having the right tools in a toolbox. It's about adding new tools when they come out. And it's about knowing how to use them. This way, you're always ready. Ready to give the best care you can.

And remember, there's a place where you can start this journey. Check out www.Caregiverstoday.org, or email us at alex@caregiverstoday.org. These websites are like a library and a classroom put together. They're full of resources, stories, and advice. You can learn a lot from them. And the best part? You can join a community of people just like you. People who care and want to learn.

Keep your mind open. Keep learning. And keep caring. With the right knowledge, you can do so much for the person who needs you. And you'll feel good about it, too. The more you know, the better you'll feel. And the better care you can give. It's a win-win all around.

Building Confidence Through Learning

You know, learning can be like a friend. It's there to help you, give you power, and make you feel strong. And when you learn about how to take care of someone with dementia, that's a big deal. It's more than just knowing things. It's about feeling sure of yourself. It's about being the best caregiver you can be. So, how does learning do all of this? Let's take a look, step by step.

First off, when you learn, you get to understand all about dementia. You find out what it's like for the person who has it. You also learn what you can do to help them. This is important because it means you can do a good job of taking care of them. You'll know what they need and how to give it to them.

Next, think about how you feel when you know something really well. You feel good, right? You feel like you can handle things. That's what happens when you learn about caregiving. You start to feel more sure of

333

yourself. And when you're sure of yourself, you do a better job. You make smarter choices. You stay calm. That's really good for you and the person you're taking care of. Now, we want you to have this kind of power. So, we've made a course. It's a course for people who take care of others. It's not a hard course. In fact, it's easy to follow. And it's full of things that you can do right away. You don't just hear about ideas—you get to use them.

Let's talk about this course. It's got nine steps. Yes, just nine. Each step is like a piece of a puzzle. When you put them all together, you see the whole picture. And each piece is easy to understand.

But that's not all. We also have a group. It's a group on Facebook. Here, you can talk to other people who are taking care of someone with dementia. It's a place where you can share your stories. You can ask questions. And you can get answers. It's like having friends who really get what you're going through.

Every month, we send out a letter. Well, it's an email, but it's like a letter. It tells you what's new. It gives you tips. Sometimes, it even tells you stories. These letters will make you feel like you're not alone. They'll remind you that you're part of a group—a group of people who care.

Now, you might be thinking, "This sounds really helpful." And it is. But we want to give you even more. So, we have a special deal. It's like getting a bunch of helpful things all at once. You can get workbooks. You can get articles that you can listen to or read. There are videos, too. And if you ever feel like you need someone to talk to, we have that as well. We can talk to you and help you find

We're here to give you what you need. And we want you to feel like you're getting something valuable. Something that makes you think, "Yes, this is good. This is what I need." That's why we do what we do.

So, let's wrap this up. Remember how we talked about learning and how it's like a friend? Well, that friend is waiting for you. It's waiting in our course, in our group, in our letters, and in all the things we offer. And all of this is there to help you build your confidence through learning.

It's time to feel good about taking care of someone with dementia. It's time to feel strong and ready for anything. And it all starts with learning. So, come join us. Let's learn together. And let's make caring for someone with dementia something we can do with confidence.

SCAN THIS AND BOOK A FREE DISCOVERY CALL NOW

Glossary Terms for Dementia Caregiving

1. **Activities of Daily Living (ADLs)** - Basic self-care tasks such as bathing, dressing, eating, and grooming that are essential for daily living.

2. **Advanced Care Planning** - Preparing for future healthcare decisions by discussing and documenting wishes with loved ones and healthcare providers.

3. **Advocacy** - The act of supporting and speaking up for the needs and rights of someone with dementia, ensuring they receive proper care and respect.

4. **Aggression** - Physical or verbal outbursts that can occur in people with dementia due to confusion, frustration, or discomfort. Managing these episodes calmly and safely is crucial.

5. **Agitation** - Restlessness and emotional distress are often observed in individuals with dementia,

338

which can be managed through calming techniques and a peaceful environment.

6. **Alzheimer's Disease** - The most common type of dementia, characterized by progressive memory loss, cognitive decline, and behavioral changes.

7. **Anticipatory Grief** - The feelings of loss and sadness that caregivers experience as they witness the gradual decline of their loved one with dementia.

8. **Bathing Assistance** - Helping a person with dementia bathe safely and comfortably, often using tools like shower chairs or hand-held showerheads to ensure ease and safety.

9. **Behavioral and Psychological Symptoms of Dementia (BPSD)**

- Non-cognitive symptoms like aggression, depression, anxiety, and hallucinations associated with dementia.

10. **Care Coordination** - Organizing and managing various aspects of a person's care, including medical appointments, medications, and support services.

11. **Caregiver Burden** - The emotional, physical, and financial strain experienced by caregivers, which can be managed through support groups, respite care, and self-care practices.

12. **Caregiver Fatigue** - Extreme tiredness and exhaustion that comes from the physical and emotional demands of caring for someone with dementia. It is important to rest and seek support to avoid burnout.

13. **Caregiver Support Groups** - Groups where caregivers can share experiences, gain emotional support, and learn from others facing similar challenges.

14. **Caregiver Stress** - The physical and emotional strain caregivers experience from the demands of caring for someone with dementia, which can lead to burnout if not managed properly.

15. **Caring Touch** - Using gentle, reassuring physical touch to comfort and calm a person with dementia, promoting connection and reducing anxiety.

16. **Cognitive Stimulation** - Activities that encourage thinking, memory, and problem-solving, such as puzzles, games, and reminiscence, which can help maintain cognitive function.

17. **Communication Techniques** - Methods used to improve communication with a person with dementia, such as speaking slowly, using simple

sentences, maintaining eye contact, and being patient.

18. **Companion Care** - Providing social interaction, support, and companionship to a person with dementia to help them feel connected and less isolated.

19. **Compassion Fatigue** - The emotional exhaustion that caregivers may feel from the constant caregiving role, which can be alleviated through self-care and seeking support.

20. **Compassionate Listening** - Fully focusing, understanding, and responding empathetically to a person with dementia, validating their feelings and experiences.

21. **Cues** - Visual or verbal reminders used to help a person with dementia remember tasks or routines, like labeling drawers or using pictures.

22. **Decision-Making Support** - Assisting a person with dementia in making decisions about their

care, respecting their autonomy and preferences as much as possible.

23. **Dementia-Friendly Environment** - An environment designed to support the needs of people with dementia, minimizing confusion and promoting independence through clear signage, good lighting, and safe spaces.

24. **Dignity** - The right of people with dementia to be treated with respect and honor, recognizing their value as individuals regardless of their cognitive abilities.

25. **Disorientation** - Confusion about time, place, or person, often seen in people with dementia, leading to feelings of being lost or unsure.

26. **Dressing Assistance** - Helping a person with dementia choose appropriate clothing and get dressed. Simplifying choices and using clothing with easy fastenings can make this task easier.

27. **Emotional Support** - Providing comfort, understanding, and encouragement to a person with dementia or a caregiver, helping them cope with their feelings and challenges.

28. **Environmental Modifications** - Changes made to the home or living space to make it safer and more comfortable for a person with dementia, such as removing tripping hazards, using nightlights, or labeling drawers.

29. **Exercise** - Physical activity that helps maintain physical health, improve mood, and reduce agitation in people with dementia. Caregivers should encourage safe, enjoyable exercises like walking or stretching.

30. **Family Counseling** - Therapy that helps family members understand dementia, cope with their emotions, and learn effective caregiving strategies.

31. **Feeding Assistance** - Helping a person with dementia eat, which might include cutting food

into smaller pieces, providing finger foods, or gently reminding them to chew and swallow.

32. **Geriatric Care Manager** - A professional who helps families coordinate and manage the care of their elderly loved ones, offering advice, and arranging necessary services.

33. **Hallucinations** - Seeing, hearing, or experiencing things that are not there, common in some types of dementia. Understanding and calmly addressing these experiences can help reduce anxiety.

34. **Hospice Care** - A type of care focused on providing comfort and support to individuals with terminal illnesses, including advanced dementia, and their families.

35. **Incontinence** - The loss of bladder or bowel control, a common issue in the later stages of dementia. Using protective pads, scheduled bathroom trips, and monitoring fluid intake can help manage this.

36. **Life Story Work** - A therapeutic activity where the person with dementia shares their life experiences to help maintain a sense of identity and improve well-being.

37. **Managing Medications** - Ensuring that a person with dementia takes their prescribed medications correctly, often requiring reminders, organizing pills, or direct supervision.

38. **Memory Aids** - Tools like calendars, clocks, and labeled items that help people with dementia remember essential information and maintain independence.

39. **Memory Care** - Specialized care for individuals with memory impairments like dementia or Alzheimer's, often provided in dedicated facilities or units.

40. **Mindfulness** - A practice that involves focusing on the present moment, which can help caregivers manage stress and connect more deeply with the person they are caring for.

41. **Mobility Support** - Assisting a person with dementia in moving around safely, which can include using mobility aids like walkers or canes or helping them navigate stairs and uneven surfaces.

42. **Music Therapy** - Using music to promote emotional well-being, reduce anxiety, and improve mood in people with dementia. Listening to familiar songs can often evoke positive memories.

43. **Nutrition Management** - Ensuring a person with dementia has a balanced diet, including healthy meals and snacks, monitoring their eating habits, and encouraging hydration.

44. **Occupational Therapy** - Therapy that helps individuals with dementia maintain independence in daily activities by adapting tasks and environments to their needs.

45. **Orientation** - Helping a person with dementia stay aware of time, place, and person, often through daily routines and familiar objects.

46. **Pain Management** - Recognizing and managing pain in a person with dementia, which might not always be communicated verbally but can be indicated through behaviors like restlessness or aggression.

47. **Personal Care** - Assisting with activities that are necessary for daily living, such as bathing, grooming, dressing, and toileting, while maintaining the person's dignity and comfort.

48. **Person-Centered Care** - An approach to care for those who respect and value the individuality of a person with dementia, focusing on their personal history, preferences, and needs.

49. **Pet Therapy** - Interaction with animals to provide comfort, reduce anxiety, and promote positive emotional experiences for people with dementia.

50. **Respite Care** - Temporary relief for caregivers, providing them a break while ensuring the person with dementia is cared for. This can help prevent caregiver burnout.

51. **Routine Establishment** - Creating a consistent daily routine to help a person with dementia feel secure and reduce confusion. Routines can include regular mealtimes, activities, and rest periods.

52. **Safety Measures** - Steps taken to protect a person with dementia from accidents and injuries, such as installing grab bars in the bathroom, using nonslip mats, or securing sharp objects and medications out of reach.

53. **Sensory Stimulation** - Activities that engage the senses, such as listening to music, touching textured objects, or smelling familiar scents, which can help people with dementia feel more connected and calmer.

54. **Sundowning** - Increased confusion and agitation occurring in the late afternoon or evening in dementia patients. Maintaining a calm environment and reducing stimuli can help manage these behaviors.

55. **Supportive Communication** - Using techniques that support understanding and connection, such as simplifying language, being patient, and using non-verbal cues like facial expressions and gestures.

56. **Team Approach** - Collaborating with a group of healthcare professionals, family members, and caregivers to provide comprehensive care for a person with dementia.

57. **Therapeutic Lying** - A technique where caregivers might use "white lies" or agree with false beliefs to avoid distress and maintain calmness in a person with dementia.

58. **Time-Outs for Caregivers** - Short breaks that caregivers take throughout the day to rest and recharge, which are crucial for preventing burnout and maintaining their own health.

59. **Validation Therapy** - A method of communicating with dementia patients that focuses on empathy and understanding, accepting their feelings and experiences rather than correcting them.

60. **Verbal Redirecting** - Gently steering a person with dementia away from a distressing topic or behavior by redirecting their attention to something more pleasant or neutral.

61. **Visual Cues** - Using pictures, symbols, or signs to help a person with dementia understand their environment and communicate more effectively.

62. **Walking Programs** - Regular, supervised walks that provide exercise and stimulation for people with dementia, helping maintain mobility and reduce agitation.

63. **Wandering** - A common behavior in dementia patients where they walk or move about without a clear destination or purpose, sometimes due to restlessness or confusion.

64. **Wandering Prevention** - Strategies to prevent a person with dementia from wandering off, such as using door alarms, wearable GPS devices, or creating safe walking paths.

65. **Wellness Checks** - Regular check-ins to ensure the person with dementia is safe, healthy, and well-cared for, often involving assessments of physical and emotional well-being.

66. **Yoga for Caregivers** - Gentle yoga exercises that caregivers can do to relieve stress, improve flexibility, and promote relaxation, supporting their overall well-being.

67. **Zoning Out** - A phenomenon where a person with dementia might appear disconnected or lost in thought, often a normal part of the condition. Gentle engagement can help bring them back to the present.

68. **Zone Therapy** - A self-care practice for caregivers that involves techniques like reflexology or massage to relieve stress and promote relaxation.

69. **Zzz Therapy** - Prioritizing sleep hygiene for both caregivers and those with dementia to ensure

restorative rest, which is crucial for emotional and physical health.

70. **Zen Moments** - Short periods of quiet reflection or meditation that caregivers and those with dementia can use to find calm and reduce anxiety, promoting a peaceful caregiving environment.

Here's a sample template for a Daily Care Log that caregivers can use to track the care and well-being of dementia patients. It provides a comprehensive structure for daily caregiving activities, helping ensure consistent care and clear communication among caregivers.

Daily Care Log

Date:_____ Patient's Name: __

Caregiver's Name: _____

---

1. **Morning Care**

   - **Wake-Up Time:** _

   - **Morning Hygiene (Brushing, Bathing, Dressing):** _

     o Time: __

     o Notes: __

   - **Breakfast:**

     o Time: __

     o Food Eaten: __

- o Fluids Taken: _

- o Notes: __

- **Morning Medication:**

  - o Time: __

  - o Medications Given: _

  - o Notes/Side Effects: __

---

2. **Midday Care**

- **Lunch:**

  - o Time: __

  - o Food Eaten: __

  - o Fluids Taken: _

  - o Notes: __

- **Midday Medication:**

  o Time: _____

  o Medications Given: _____

  o Notes/Side Effects: _____

- **Afternoon Activities:**

  o Type: _____

  o Time: _____

  o Notes:_____

---

3. **Evening Care**

   - **Dinner:**

     o Time: __

     o Food Eaten: __

     o Fluids Taken: _

     o Notes: __

- **Evening Medication:**

  o Time: __

  o Medications Given: _

  o Notes/Side Effects: _

- **Evening Activities:**

  o Type: __

  o Time: __

  o Notes: _

---

4. **Night Care**

- **Bedtime Routine:**

  o Time: __

  o Activities (Toileting, Teeth Brushing, etc.): ___

  o Notes: _

- **Sleep Time:** ____
- **Nighttime Observations:**
  - o Wake-ups/Restlessness: ___
  - o Notes: _

---

5. **Behavior & Mood Tracking**
- **General Mood:**
  - o Morning: _____
  - o Afternoon: ___
  - o Evening: _____
- **Behavioral Observations:**
  - o Notable Behaviors: _
  - o Possible Triggers: ___
  - o Caregiver Response: _____

6. Additional Notes/Concerns

_____

_____

_____

Caregiver Signature: _____

Date: __

CAREGIVERS
TRAINING

End Caregiver Stress

FEELING OVERWHELMED?

TIRED?

DISCOVER HOW TO TURN THESE CHALLENGES INTO EMPOWERMENT

This course isn't just about care – it's about revolutionizing your approach, mastering stress management, and reigniting your passion.

Each step is a leap towards not just surviving, but thriving in your caregiving role. And the best part?

You'll gain the skills to teach and inspire others, creating a ripple effect of positive change. Don't wait for burnout to take over. Take control, transform your caregiving journey, and become an empowered leader in your community.

ENROLL NOW AND START YOUR PATH TO EMPOWERMENT AND RESILIENCE TODAY!

For More Information ,Contact Us

alex@caregiverstoday.org

www.caregiverstoday.org

CAREGIVERS TODAY